MASTERY
OF THE TRUE SELF

The Discipline of Love Through
Sadhana, Aradhana & Prabhupati

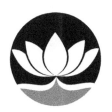

SADHANA SINGH

© 2021 Kundalini Research Institute
Published by the Kundalini Research Institute
Training • Publishing • Research • Resources
PO Box 1819
Santa Cruz, NM 87532
www.kundaliniresearchinstitute.org

ISBN: 978-1-940837-41-3

Managing Editor: HariShabd Kaur (Mariana Lage)

Line Editor: Siri Neel Kaur Khalsa

Associate Line Editor: Shanti Kaur Khalsa

Consulting Editor: Nirvair Singh Khalsa and Amrit Singh Khalsa

Proofreading: Sangeet Kaur Khalsa

Reviewer: Siri Neel Kaur Khalsa and Padmani Kaur

Translator: Giovanna Ruiu and Susan Duncan

Design and Layout: Prana Projects (Ditta Khalsa, Biljana Nedelkovska)

Photography: Dham Khalsa Photography

Models: Dasha Mays, Eddie Castro, Edmund Miera (Deg Raj Singh), Elaine Bressler, Eva Vai, Lakshmi Kaur Khalsa, Sat Darshan Kaur Khalsa, Sat Sandesh Kaur and Sukh Meher Kaur

The diet, exercise and lifestyle suggestions in this book come from ancient yogic traditions. Nothing in this book should be construed as medical advice. Any recipes mentioned herein may contain potent herbs, botanicals and naturally occurring ingredients which have traditionally been used to support the structure and function of the human body. Always check with your personal physician or licensed health care practitioner before making any significant modification in your diet or lifestyle, to ensure that the ingredients or lifestyle changes are appropriate for your personal health condition and consistent with any medication you may be taking. For more information about Kundalini Yoga as taught by Yogi Bhajan® please see www.yogibhajan.org and www.kundaliniresearchinstitute.org.

This publication has received the KRI Seal of Approval. This Seal is given only to products that have been reviewed for accuracy and integrity of the sections containing the 3HO lifestyle and Kundalini Yoga as taught by Yogi Bhajan®.

DEDICATION

In memory of my teacher, Yogi Bhajan,
whose light and wisdom has guided my life.

To my sons, Japji Singh and Sukh Anand Singh,
and all the children of the next generation.

ONG NAMO GURU DEV NAMO

I bow to the Divine Teacher
who is within me

TABLE OF CONTENTS

3. ARADHANA

INTRODUCTION

The book you have in your hands is the compilation of four different essays based on my own practical experience of Kundalini Yoga, integrating Yogi Bhajan's teachings throughout a period that spans over half my lifetime. In particular, these four texts cover an 18-year time frame starting from the year 2000. They explore the most adventurous experience of human evolution of recognizing, accepting, integrating, and expressing the self.

During that same period, as a part of my research, I wrote 10 other books and essays, which consolidated my study. This entire process deepened my understanding of the phases leading to mastery of the self, and resulted in the compilation you are now reading.

For thousands of years, students, yogis, and sages have practiced self-inquiry by exploring every aspect of consciousness that serves to awaken the self, reveal the authentic nature of the spirit, and transform subconscious habits and preconceptions that distract from recognizing our true inner identity. It is an inquiry that advanced the development of a common path, through which the self can find its way through blocks and challenges.

This journey allows us to consciously and naturally discover our true Selves. By setting our qualities and potential to the service of the time and space in which we live, our Self can manifest and radiate. The totality of this legacy of research is contained within the technology of Kundalini Yoga as taught by Yogi Bhajan®, which, as a 'science of the Self,' offers us the way to be human.

This 'science of Self' known as Humanology, is an empirical science that allows us to understand the applied psychology and dynamics of our growth and life cycles. A sutra in the ancient yogic scriptures describes three parts to this process: *Sadhana*, *Aradhana*, and *Prabhupati*. *Sadhana* is itself the discipline, *Aradhana* is the assimilation of that discipline, and *Prabhupati* is the crystallization of that discipline. These three masteries outline the possible progression to attain our mission in this life – finding the Infinite within our power and fullness in our everyday life.

Humanology, clarifies the methodological progression of the Self on life's journey. The order of progression is crucial. Frustration, error, and pain in our lives come if we allow ignorance to guide us. When we allow ourselves to be seduced by easy shortcuts or fear of facing reality, we go against our true nature, alienating ourselves from the harmony that surrounds us. This same process intensified my relationship with Yogi Bhajan and gradually helped me understand his state of awareness, reading his teachings in the light of the essence and spirit of human potential, rather than technically or philosophically.

The process of *Sadhana*, *Aradhana*, and *Prabhupati* restores a person's awareness of their essence, thanks to the awakening and practical use of the projective meditative mind. Mastery requires an appropriate state of consciousness to move through the teachings with a flow of awareness. Experience then naturally occurs on the basis of reality.

Therefore, this book intends to facilitate the process of self-mastery through a progressive understanding of the teachings – and consequentially to pave the way for others to experience this same process. Through this real experience, the continuity of the teachings may be maintained, which would otherwise risk disappearance without the embodied continuation of human transmission. Ultimately, the only absolute priority is to remember that the power of the human spirit remains indomitable.

Without a process of integrating the Self into the practicalities of life, we can easily confuse the purpose of life itself with the means to achieving it, seeking satisfaction and happiness in the instruments and not in the goal. Mastery is the very goal itself – it does not lie in gratification received from objects, situations, or people, but rather in how these relationships are managed.

From this real, altruistic, and loving perspective, a concrete goal emerges in which our authenticity can express itself by serving your mission's uniqueness. We can call it 'being effective,' a term that may seem rather cold. Yet, it is a unique human priority; it allows us to express our original creative matrix by playing and serving our precise and irreplaceable role in the ordered chaos of the universe. This is life.

We are effective when our awareness keeps intact the essence of our intention, which our Self has committed to embrace as our mission. *Sadhana* arouses and re-awakens us to who we are by revealing our deep intent. *Aradhana* consolidates the clarity of commitment and strengthens our motivation and determination by aligning our inner intention with our external projection. *Prabhupati* integrates the delivery of our Self and, therefore, the fulfillment of our destiny.

The process of integrating the spirit is this - it is straightforward: There is no right or wrong; there are only differences. There is no extreme in polarities or the will to solve them. Instead, the process focuses on managing the polarities with grace, without 'maybe's,' 'buts' or 'I don't knows' - simply in unity with the Self that animates us. Otherwise, it is impossible to find meaning in life.

Integrating the spirit is a simple process of becoming an expert of the Self, identified as excellence. Without consistent and progressive experience in these three phases of spiritual discipline, we remain victims of a circumstantial reality hidden within ourselves. Becoming aware of this concealed inner agenda, accepting it, and transforming it, is the most satisfying rebirth.

The experience gained from the emancipation from our seemingly inescapable inner saboteur reveals intrinsic potential. It aligns our psyche with the teachings, naturally becoming a flow of love and hope - an audible and synchronized vibratory frequency. But this can only occur if we dare to explore our unknown infinite nature. Once we consolidate this process, we become invincible. The circumstances are no longer relevant because we have already won over our unconscious and subconscious nonsense and have found victory itself.

Finally, I would like to share five guidelines to mastery. Yogi Bhajan condensed the complex transformational process of mastery into these practical concepts. I will resist the temptation to explore them in detail here, so that you can read about them in the following chapters. Practice and experiment, go within and be, keep up, project, and deliver yourself so that you can enjoy them in your own way.

Guidelines to Mastery

1. To be a leader, lead by example.

2. Serve the mission, not the self.

3. To lead, adopt all practical roles, so people will believe in you.

4. Learn to have mastery through the example of a master – the perfect student becomes the perfect master.

5. With courage, serve impeccably with absolute sacrifice of the self.

Sat Naam
Sadhana Singh
July 24, 2019

DISCIPLINE

THE ART OF LOVING

The evolutionary process of human life is to become ourselves, complete and competent. We can see this progression as awakening and transforming. In Kundalini Yoga, the three stages of spiritual development are *Sadhana, Aradhana,* and *Prabhupati*.

Sadhana is our daily spiritual discipline. In *sadhana*, we awake and perceive our essence – the spirit that animates us – and vibrate a deep sense of belonging to the Infinite. In *Sadhana*, we accept this love affair with God, as a bride accepts her husband. In *Aradhana*, we experience love and longing for the Divine in the depth of our being. The marriage takes place, with all the joys and crises of shared life. By discipline and endurance, we overcome the crises dispelling the sense of separation from the Beloved. In a state of a complete merger, we feel the excellence of unconditional love. This is *Prabhupati*.

Being ourselves is the core for our expansion and the fulcrum around which to rotate. Expressing and delivering ourselves is a manifestation on the material plane of our spirit and essence. As human beings, we live successful lives when we are complete and when our electromagnetic field radiates. The process of being successful implies exposing ourselves to life completely. This brings multiplication and intensification of interactions, greater complexity in managing the energetic and material fruits we have attracted, and greater choices regarding possibilities and responsibilities.

New challenges will manifest along the journey towards wholeness of being– this is natural and necessary. Without challenges, life is unable to provide the opportunities to elevate our values and discover our virtues and resources. This process makes us competent. Every action creates friction and tension, and every action has the potential to release friction and tension. Simply being alive creates encounters and consequences that multiply as we expand and become more complete. However, as we expand, if we lose touch with our true Self, then the challenges become more complex, and the ways to overcome them become more tortuous. Our outer progress generates an inner regression. To avoid this regression, we must maintain a solid balance in the three realms of having, being, and becoming and equalize the expansion of our mental and spiritual paths. This marks the difference between a life simply lived and a life expressed in the complete knowledge of ourselves. Consistency with our true Self gives us satisfaction, and discipline allows us to expand while remaining constant within.

I include this quote from Yogi Bhajan that inspired my work and specifically this section of the book:

The price of nobility is discipline. The price of ecstasy is Sadhana. The price of God is living without doubt.[1]

Nobility is the radiance of spirit that expresses itself in life. It maintains its intentions, words, and actions at a high frequency, to honor not an illusionary status but instead the character of excellence. The result is a code of conduct that keeps us from being corrupt and betraying our true identity. Nobility is the condition through which we maintain the human essence of sovereignty. Ultimately, nobility places a person above any situation, guiding them to elevate others.

Nobility gives us the ability to forgive the unforgivable, accept the unacceptable, and forget the unforgettable. It is a path to freedom – once we have reached that altitude, we can see what was invisible and hear what was previously inaudible. Discipline is key to nobility defining the guidelines we choose to follow daily to refine our projection.

Ecstasy is a precise, unambiguous condition. It occurs when our level of intimacy with ourselves is so deep that it enables us to rejoice and enjoy ourselves. Ecstasy is sublime, intoxicating, and real. The Greeks coined this word by putting together *Ek*, which stands for "out," and *stasis*, which means "staying," or "state." Thus, ecstasy means "out of the normal state" of doing and thinking. Here, we identify with the spirit that illuminates and exalts, giving us a sense of accomplishment

---

[1] Yogi Bhajan, March 20, 1985

as human beings. We are in ecstasy when the flow of thought stops and the veil of maya, which creates separation and deception, lifts. From the window of our mind, we see our soul, and we merge with everything. The price to pay to reach this state of ecstasy and nobility is *Sadhana*. In fact, without opening the chakras and cleansing the subconscious through meditation, we will not have nobility. Without the experience of ecstasy, we will not realize our spirit.

God is the energy of the Infinite – immeasurable and indefinable. It is everywhere and in every part of us. We nourish a strong sense of belonging to this creative energy, even when we are not always aware of it. In truth, we perceive God when we are in contact with our soul and cease experiencing duality. Then we go from divided to divine, from unidirectional to all-encompassing, distracted to attentive, dispersed to contained, wanting to be liked to appreciating others, insecure to confident, controlling to containing, and from complaining to happiness. We know God when we unite our inner self and His soul, like a drop of water united in the ocean. When we sacrifice doubt, the experience of God within us makes us become like Him.

In the teachings, three concepts describe our relationship to actions: *karam, dharam* and *param*. *Karma* is the consequences of past actions that reproduce repetitive dynamics that we may see and reconcile. Mindlessly pursuing *karmic* tendencies equates to becoming a victim of fate. Until we resolve our karma, we remain stagnate and do not evolve. *Dharma* is righteousness in action. It dissolves karma and is the most direct path to reach our destiny. *Param* is doubt, the duality between being and non-being, love and fear, and therefore between *karma* and *dharma*.

Discipline is our applied *dharma*. *Sadhana* is how we burn karma. The experience of God is when we dispel doubt. Love is our path once we pay the price of discipline and resolve our duality to reach our destiny. Being ourselves, complete and competent, we understand love and we educate ourselves to love unconditionally.

Doubt and duality are the antitheses of love. Discipline is the portal of love. *Sadhana* is the progression of love. Kundalini Yoga is the science of the Self, raising our awareness in direct proportion to our capacity to love. Therefore, our only goal is to love.

It is true that love is a gift. It cannot be forced; it can only be accepted and then expanded and balanced. Love has no limits because it is a concept that belongs to the Unknown. It is not restricted to our feelings, emotions, or desires. We place our trust in something with no guarantee. We simply trust and open our hearts toward others or ourselves without thought of value. Who deserves hatred? No one does. It is not that we do not suffer. It is not that we do not experience pain, but instead, love dissolves these experiences as an ongoing process. That is why love is blind and asks no questions. If the subconscious is full of garbage, we will not achieve this state of acceptance. We may meet love but cannot contain it. If we cannot accept all that may come, our love will remain incomplete and consume our hearts with grievances, regrets and guilt.

Love that flows brings blessings to whoever perceives it. However, to experience this state of ecstasy we must have reached and digested its opposite. To live from the spirit, with the spirit, and for the spirit, we must have experienced desperation without spirit. Love will bring prosperity because this is the language of the Infinite.

Through our perceptual and sensory skills in this finite existence, love creates the experience of the Infinite and it materializes it into knowledge. The human being's creative capacity to make the impossible possible is love. Discipline creates the conditions, the entirety of the human psychic sphere so that love may blow through it like a fresh breeze. It is an intangible perception, a faint feeling of an infinitesimal tinge of love, a fraction of a memory inherent in us. This glimmer is enough to motivate our discipline to reach a permanent and profound understanding of our spirit, others, and life that without love makes no sense.

Relationship through the lens of Patanjali's Eight Limbs

Kundalini Yoga recognizes the essence and process of yoga's evolution in the reflective writings of Patanjali who meticulously analyzed the structure and outcome of the discipline of yoga in the Eight Limbs. They are "limbs," not steps, as they are not progressive stages but dependent on the practitioner's individual growth in varying proportions. The first two limbs are *yama* and *niyama*: the ethical discipline of the do's and do not's. They are followed by asana, the physical postures, *praanayama*, techniques for control of vital energy, *Pratyaharaa*, withdrawal of attention from external senses, *dharana*, focused concentration, *dhyana*, deep meditation and samadhi, contemplation or union with the Divine.

We can apply the Eight Limbs to understand the relationships and the art of loving. *Yama* and *niyama*, the basic requirements of not harming others or ourselves, is a fundamental requirement of love. Without these guidelines, even if we begin a relationship with good intentions, we undermine it with negative and impulsive actions that distort the relationship's reality. They influence how complete we are, how open we are to each other, and how willing we are to explore new paths.

In *Asana*, we face the relationship and the posture we adopt towards the other person. How we wish to be seen by others – noble or hidden, vital or depressed, the roles we are willing to take, what pressure we are willing to tolerate, and how much grace and continuity we maintain with the other person.

Praanayama is how we communicate, assimilate, and integrate within a relationship. It is the exchange of vital energy with others in verbal and physical interaction. *Praanayama* is the experience of breathing the same air, of breathing in others until we are in each other's cells.

In *Pratyaharaa*, we recognize that the other person is a gift from the Infinite, as we are for them. It is understanding

6

the principle that when two people connect, they grow and evolve exponentially. The other person is the spirit of the universe and reminds us that we are also the universe's spirit. In *Pratyaharaa*, the true nature of the soul becomes tangible.

Dharana is the unilateral state of concentration where the gaze of awareness focuses on the other, and in return, their gaze is fixed on us. The experience becomes intense. Along with the wonder of the visible beauty, the mind colors the experience with contrasts and friction, resistance and doubt, a flurry of impulses that the human being contains in the meditative process. The relationship becomes exactly that, a meditation.

In *Dhyana*, we are so mutual that we no longer perceive the relationship as external; the other no longer seems separate. If we maintain this state long enough to become stable and unquestionable, we enter into Samadhi, and the two beings become one, merged in the ecstasy of transcendent love.

From Patanjali's viewpoint, yoga is life itself, with the same goals and highest values to nurture excellence in everything. Sometimes we try to protect ourselves from love, from its unknown variables and risky consequences, while the only possible protection lies in opening ourselves entirely to love. Any other attempt is counterproductive for us and others.

Kundalini Yoga as a Tool

Discipline is nothing more than mastery of a particular set of elements. We submit to discipline to evoke an opening to find the right answer and a better understanding. All the required resources are already within us. It is just a matter of finding the right combination. Discipline connects us to these aspects. For this reason, we practice Kundalini Yoga kriyas that clear our subconscious and end its release of thoughts, fears, and impulses.

Regular exposure to something gives us expertise, whether it is a topic, a skill, or a human characteristic. Our adult life reveals what we experienced in our childhood and our childhood reveals what we experienced in the womb. As adults, we have a choice, either relate to our environment or disconnect from it. Through discipline, we consciously decide what areas to relate to or not.

Essentially, first, we have to reveal ourselves inward to the light of the Soul and only then can we radiate outward. We must discipline ourselves to be inwardly vulnerable, and then we can expose ourselves to outward experiences, staying in reality and contemplating it in the present. Discipline is educating ourselves to be what we were born to be. Our ignorance, our avoidance of reality, creates what we perceive to be tragedies that we experience.

We need intention and commitment in order to grow. There is no intention without attention, and without attention, our intention is at risk. As we have seen, our subconscious projections and fears may influence our intentions. However, we know without fear our intention is accurate and why we need to clear the subconscious of all fear.

Knowing ourselves requires fearless discipline - to assess and evaluate ourselves under pressure. Often anxiety creates moments of attraction or repulsion and we are tempted to replace the uncomfortable feelings with momentary feelings of satisfaction or relief. Instead, if we stop and observe, staying in the intensity of the feeling, we discover our strengths. It may be that what drives us to react is the guard-dog, our subconscious. We may find that we do not die by stopping but instead discover our inner Self's resources and get to know ourselves more deeply.

Devoid of urgency and in search of reality, discipline identifies the cause that has produced a dysfunction as either an effect or consequence. Containing and elevating ourselves, we can look at the situation from a different context and another state of consciousness. We can observe the situation without reacting to it and transform it. Attention, discipline's companion, when compromised, requires a strong established relationship with the Self to come back. This relationship requires time to learn and observe through tolerance.

There are three stages of evolution in consciousness that support each other and that are interactive and progressive. The first realm is that of needs, the essential experiential realm of the instinctual self. In this stage, it is critical to understand the balance between what is needed and what is believed to be necessary, what is an actual priority and the "never enough" syndrome. The second realm is that of being – just experiencing ourselves in the heart's integrity and innocence. There is neither drama nor originality in being, just ourselves resting in our own presence. The third realm is that of becoming – where our integrity explores and delivers itself in continuous change; the essence and identity remain while in a constant search for what is not yet known.

How can we become if we are not? How can we be if we do not have? If we can have, it means that we are. If we are, it means we can become. We can unfold in many different directions. However, every time we lose our foundation of consciousness, the next realm becomes inaccessible. If, while we are becoming, we lose contact with the being and having, we are lost and the work must start again. If we reach the desired realm and then lose our relationship with those we experienced along the way, we need to pause and rebuild our foundation.

In Kundalini Yoga, these three realms relate to the "lower triangle," which includes the first three chakras, and refers to safety, creativity, and power issues. The Heart Chakra, the fourth chakra, represents the transition from "me" to "we." Lastly, the "upper triangle" includes the fifth, sixth and seventh chakras and relates sequentially to expression, intuition, and knowledge.

"Having, being, and becoming" describe the lower triangle, heart center, and upper triangle. The active interplay between these realms is the flow of consciousness. The shift in consciousness weaves and blends these three realms, creating conditions for the spirit to prevail. Discipline is necessary, so that the spirit penetrates all three realms and can be experienced. Discipline is a constant process of cleansing the subconscious, a continuous and progressive commitment to exposing ourselves to our spirit's subtlety and our relationship to the Infinite. Discipline is a revolutionary and evolutionary movement to rebel against the slavery that our ego and intellect inflict upon us. When we break these bonds, no one can manipulate or control us.

Symbolically, this process has been represented and taught in most spiritual disciplines as *surrendering* – giving our head to God and keeping our heart attached to the Infinite. The further we dwell in discipline, the more we realize that practice is not an end in itself; it serves a greater purpose. The goal is not the discipline for itself but the application of caliber, that we obtain through our practice, to achieve the impossible. Caliber is the ability to hold steady and make sense of what has lost all sense, the ability to maintain our authority in relation to what we are committed to honoring. Without self-authority, supported by caliber – the unknown authority, the subconscious guides our lives. This permits us to develop and transform ourselves with graceful authority, bringing the psyche to realize and fulfill our Self.

In our rush to grow up, many of us did not take the time to realize our spirit. We may be effective and able to achieve something, but it is a compensation for our inability to be and know ourselves. Our rush to become something is often an escape from being and having, an attempt to cover up what we do not want to face and ultimately accept.

Most of the things we do, the commitments we make, and the distortions we allow ourselves to have, are an attempt to compensate for the feelings of inadequacy that we have towards ourselves. Discomfort, the primary anxiety created by the simple act of being alive, occupies every moment of our time and influences our actions. The human being has always known this dysfunction and has perpetually tried to make up for it. Life today offers a multitude of distractions focusing us on the outside and obstructing us from ourselves. This, coupled with the speed with which time moves, makes us split from ourselves and easily anesthetizes us to our inner feelings. It is irrelevant whether we suffer or are happy because, in the end, we are sedating ourselves with the drug of doing. The compulsion of doing distracts us and temporarily soothes us from the reality of being. It calms the fear that we do not have the strength or tolerance to integrate the aspects of ourselves.

It is a well-masked process, and we are only aware of a small part of it. When we stop doing what we have always done, we drop the mask. If we control the impulsive reactions and the emotions that they trigger, we can dwell in pure existence. When we flee from ourselves, non-action is an abyss inhabited by monsters. When we acknowledge ourselves, that void is our totality, from which we regenerate and create.

Mechanical doing, occupying every space and time with activity exemplified by the need to learn as much information as possible and to be connected to everything beyond what is necessary, is a way to prove our existence – prove we are alive. When we escape from ourselves and act purely from the fear of not doing, we postpone the natural confrontation with ourselves. We avoid taking responsibility for ourselves and create an alternative, unreal lifestyle built on doing. Any achievement gained has no roots, no foundation, and is thus ephemeral and unsatisfactory.

The only real thing is the Self. To be true in this existence, we have to be ourselves. If we are not ourselves, we are not in touch with reality. Therefore, anything we relate to will be unreal; nothing we build is elevating and, thus, cannot bring happiness.

Real-life is acting reliably with our selves and not reacting to what we do not want to accept. Life is to act dependably and in favor of our Self. Life's specific purpose is to serve, using our qualities and abilities to deliver ourselves' integrity and essence. Taking action to avoid facing our fears, strengths, or inconsistencies means not allowing ourselves to learn about ourselves because behind these uncomfortable facets of ourselves lies our unique creative potential. If we apply discipline to act in favor of our Self, regardless of what this entails, we distinguish our Self from the shadow self, with its polarities and reactions. The path that leads to this includes tolerance and ultimately brings us to a state of neutrality and non-discrimination. Here, there is no intellectual reasoning and no emotional evaluation. We naturally grasp the meaning of ourselves, and we naturally realize ourselves.

Kundalini Yoga originates as a tool to discipline ourselves to be our self, giving us an altitude that allows us to recognize the real from the fake and an attitude to process and include rather than deny and avoid. It arouses awareness and orchestrates personal dynamics to reveal our inner and outer reality. It is a straightforward discipline because it quickly leads us to be what, in truth, we already are. That is why we call it the Science of Reality, the Yoga of Awareness.

We see, decrypt, identify and correct the intellectual, psychological, and physical spheres through the electromagnetic field. The vibrational frequency expressed in the electromagnetic field shows how the life force and the psyche flow freely within our being, resulting in its radiance. This flow and its energetic vibration can expand in proportion to our psychic blocks' decrease, thereby demonstrating our inner conflict or our inner harmony. Thus, the magnetic field testifies to an internal state of fear or love, contraction or expansion, orbit or consistency. Exposure to the yogic techniques, as numerous as the basic psychophysical human needs, corrects the dysfunctions that occur in each of us, using the physical body to restore the proper flow in the electromagnetic field that, consequently, affects the psyche.

The technology of Kundalini Yoga is concentrated in kriyas. A kriya is a sequence of postures (*asanas*), combined with hand positions (*mudras*), concentration of the eyes (*dhristi*), specific breathing techniques (*praanayama*), and certain frequencies of sound (*mantra*). Together it stimulates the physical, mental, and energetic systems. It is a complete action with specific practice times, pauses, and relaxations resulting in a predictable and desired state of consciousness.

The subconscious decisively has an impact on the body to stimulate the electromagnetic field. The action of the kriya diagonally penetrates the subconscious to remove the blocks that inhibit our ability to relate to something. It educates the neurons to find new associative paths, unraveling old habitual patterns, and opening new opportunities and scenarios.

Kundalini Yoga combines the functional and impersonal minds to interact in specific proportions to experience new mental habits appropriate for every kind of need, task, and situation. Perceptive and creative activity is improved and refined with meditation and the vibration of the sound current, stimulating the hypothalamus, thalamus, and frontal lobe that are responsible for the development of our self-sensory system. In the future, humans will fully develop this system and recognize our inner world, enabling us to be authentic in our being.

In Kundalini Yoga, the kundalini energy is stimulated to awaken and ascend. This gives clarity, awareness, and magnitude to understand ourselves and others' reality and to perceive the consequences of our intentions, words, and actions. The physical body mirrors the acceleration in awareness, by strengthening the nervous and glandular systems to support and regulate all the other systems. Health and vitality enable us to identify ourselves and then expand. It is a path to self-love and love for others, for life, and the environment.

Through meditation, the subconscious's cleansing reveals the psychic structures, with its shadow identity and hidden agenda. The activation of our frontal lobe gives us the ability to identify and constantly refine thoughts and tendencies. We achieve complete integrity of the mental body by expanding the energetic body enough to allow us to see ourselves clearly and then attain the honor of being our true Self.

A Prelude

The understanding of discipline is a prelude to exploring *Sadhana*, *Aradhana*, and *Prabhupati*. In this study, we will delve deeper into the reasons why the human being, already perfect in creation, needs discipline to experience the true self and be able to live life freely, in love and happiness.

In my experience as a teacher, I have explored the nature and methods of discipline and its technology. I am fascinated by how discipline can produce substantial, predictable, and repeatable changes in our physiological systems and consciousness. I have tried with enthusiasm to unfold the teachings to read between the lines, in the corners and triangles they employ, and the levers they use to lift the impossible. Until now, I have focused on the "how" and "what" in the realm of discipline. Our understanding is not complete unless we explore the "why." So today, I ask the unequivocal question, "Why is discipline necessary to live a conscious, healthy, and happy existence?"

When we choose discipline to avoid the present moment's discomfort, it is no different from taking an aspirin when we have a headache – we are treating the symptom. It is not a cure, but it is a start! Becoming aware of the symptom broadens our perspective. It awakens us and calls us to take time to sit and reflect upon ourselves. Starting from the symptom is like stepping into an existing story, looking at life with its trends, characteristics, and circumstances. Viewing ourselves under the lens of discipline exposes those things that do not allow us to be who we are. It does so gradually, inevitably, and precisely. Discipline is a tool for self-evaluation, self-acceptance, and self-projection.

Lacking discipline, we tend to look only on the outside, blaming the world for our own inabilities and sense of inadequacy. We want to govern the world, change it, and organize it. With discipline, we observe our inner world and separate the real from the imaginary, facilitating the understanding of the Self and experiencing how each shift in consciousness, every opening, growth, and inner revolution impacts the outside world. We recognize how sensitive the environment is and how it reflects our attitude and internal condition. When we put aside the concept of right and wrong, it helps us understand our inner reality and our projection of it to the outside world. No external situation defines our inner state, level of awareness, or degree of discipline. Still, the way we react to what happens to us is a precise diagnosis of how aware we are at that particular moment in time. If we don't have discipline, we perceive the external world as wrong. When we begin to discipline ourselves, we understand that the outside world is actually manifesting in response to our energy frequency.

We attract all that revolves around us by projecting consciously or subconsciously or a conflicted mixture of both. The frequency that we project will attract a similar or an opposite frequency. For example, occasionally, we perceive that everything seems to happen at the same time. Calamities are not accidental; we have drawn them to us. What we have attracted brings opportunities as well — we only have to be able to see them. Without discipline, calamities become oppressive burdens that we would like to escape, but we miss the opportunity by running away.

I would like to share my own experience with the phenomena of discipline. In writing my book *Everyday Excellence*[2] something remarkable happened. For the first time, I wrote without a predetermined didactic scheme. Instead, I allowed myself to tell stories, ask questions, and follow a natural path in presenting the teachings. To my delight, the writing flowed quite naturally. This opened me up to new and unexplored aspects of my creative potential and, at the same time, revealed hidden aspects of myself that I had been reluctant to bring out of the shadows. I realized that I had been maintaining an outdated stereotype that suppressed the "symptom," which was the creative tension naturally found in writing, to avoid the awareness of inner fear. Giving space to this weakness allowed me to deeply understand that the teachings were very practical and concrete to rely on in real-life experiences. Affording myself to be in that state of awareness allowed me to go deeper into my humanity and better assimilate the teachings, transforming division into unity, differentiation into uniqueness, and a stereotype into a pure state.

I would like to share with you something I wrote about three years ago:

[2] KRI, 2012

"power of projection, your self-reverence, will win over every-thing for you. This is the path to victory. There is no substitute for victory. Victory is not for others or against others, or for any material or spiritual conquest. Victory means being successful in using awareness on all the subconscious, unconscious, or semi- conscious matter. The rest is just hypocrisy and deception. You must not seek wealth, let wealth come looking for you. Do not look for victory, let victory come looking for you. If this is not your process, wealth will not flow, strength will have no source, wisdom will not have height, and your identity won't be as vast as the Infinite. Nothing can come to you without the vibratory effect of the mind. Polarity must communicate to attract. Every calamity is a test for your own reality. If you face calamities with your reality, you will win, because God will be on your side. The enemy is what you think in your mind - other than that there is no enemy. It is a limitation that you call fear. It is the shadow that you call a threat."

Reading these lines now, I recognize that we often teach with instinctive ease the topic we need to learn the most. This has a magnified impact if we also want to learn in addition to needing to learn. When we are entirely in the process of what we are teaching and living the experience, we teach with strength and confidence. When we attain this and reach mastery, we manifest excellence and evoke transcendence.

This new process led me to open up to a more complete understanding of discipline, its application and resulting consequences. The consequence of success sheds light on the depths that we did not want to explore, understand, or accept. Only by diving deeper into these depths can we maintain success bringing a large number of possibilities and relationships to be contained and nourished. It is a call to humility, which is the foundation of all excellence.

Discipline becomes *Dharma* when it is elevated above the normal sequence of action and reaction. Sometimes, in the middle of life's difficulty and complexity, the only way to continue forward is to touch rock bottom and allow a little ego-death. First, we explore, accept, and embrace the cause of pain and fear. Then, we rise above it, more complete, undamaged, aligned, powerful, and united, experiencing the incomparable satisfaction of resurrection. Numerous situations and relationships provide opportunities to live consciously and expansively through the soul. Without the guidance of the spirit and the interaction of consciousness, the mind and personality cannot contain the totality of the experience. They no longer are in reality and only try to control it, and in doing so lose the flow and potentiality of life. In essence, discipline is necessary to live in the spirit.

Life is the experience of the present moment, as it is happening, after integrating the past and investing in the future. The body is the past, the mind is the present, and the spirit is the future. Discipline is the best investment for the future – it captures the past richness and magnifies the present. Whoever you are and whatever you want to achieve, you must do it with love, drawing on the spirit's strength, depth, and neutrality. To climb up to the heights of the spirit, you must first descend into the depths of matter. Anyone who wants to experience heaven must first experience its opposite. As the ancient Native American wisdom teaches:

"Religion is for people who are afraid of going to hell.
Spirituality is for those who've already been there[3]."

[3] Often attributed to Vine Deloria, Jr.

Your Own Discipline

The word "discipline" comes from the Latin word *discere*, "to learn," and so the word "disciple" is "the one who learns." The term discipline emphasizes the formative rather than the informative aspect of learning. Knowledge is important, but not as important as the process of learning. How you learn the teachings is not as important as the fruits of the experience that come from applying their discipline to your life.

Discipline is the necessary tool for re-educating those personal tendencies that diverge from our inner nature. We discipline ourselves to be complete, consistent, and incorruptible. We expose ourselves to constant training to make our expression more effective and make the system of communication between our inner nature and the reception of external stimuli more sophisticated. We discipline ourselves to give our intentions, words, and actions an orbit, an effect, and a definite impact, to maintain the true essence of who we are and what we want.

Developing oneself is a form of training, and it requires discipline. Spiritual training must, as such, train us to have a clear and complete perception of ourselves, our circumstantial reality, and our Infinite Reality. From this state of awareness, we have a solid base from which we are able to understand, experience, and master the creative process. The science we must study and the training we must discipline ourselves in is the awareness of the Self. Each one of us is a microcosm, created in the image and likeness of the same creative matrix as the universe. Knowing from within our essence, structure, polarity, mental processes, dynamics, and tendencies, we will know the macrocosm. We will intuitively know how to relate to every situation or person and how to perceive their reality. We will, in turn, act as creative factors to realize the soul's intimate desire to manifest its purpose in relation to Infinity.

This is what the science of Kundalini Yoga provides, a way for each human being's essence and existence to connect to its infinite nature. Kundalini Yoga translates metaphysics into daily living within space and time. Therefore, we discipline ourselves to be aware. Awareness, a term that contains the meaning of reality, is a constant flow of clarity that highlights what is true. It is the compass of the soul and brings light onto reality, finding expansion toward totality. Awareness means being constantly mindful of the interaction of ourselves as a finite identity, with ourselves as an Infinite Potential Identity.

The finite identity is not inferior. It is, in fact, essential and necessary to deal with life. However, the finite identity can become a significant obstacle to expansion when its need for security drives us to act from fear, damaging others and ourselves. When it is balanced, the finite identity gives a solid foundation to the Infinite Self to be expressed in tangible and sustained happiness. Our physical structure, anatomy, physiology, and psychology are made in the Divine's image. Without the finite identity, we would not have the Infinite Identity. We would not be the manifestation on earth of the Divine Energy from where everything comes and to where it all goes back. In that polarity, the human being is the link between the cosmos and the earth.

Any innovation created, on the one hand, has marked the human being's intellectual progress and, on the other hand, has contributed to the decline of the sensory and spiritual human being. Wonderful tools have cured many diseases, released human beings and animals from performing heavy labor, and developed global communication that, in turn, have contributed to the development of society. At the same time, though, the unbalanced use of advanced technology has sedated our intuitive ability for guidance and movement. It has made our systems and physiological faculties lazy, lowering our vitality, health, and perception standards. The unbalanced use of these technologies has dramatically reduced our ability to discipline ourselves.

Like everything else in nature, the body and the psyche operate in such a way that, when certain capacities or systems are not used over a certain period of time, the pranic and physiological intelligence focus on other capabilities, nourishing and investing in different actions or intentions.

Let us observe plants, trees, flowers, and fruits. They can be delicious, healing, or poisonous. Each plant has its odor, color, taste, texture and function. Likewise, qualities and tendencies differ in human beings. Everything is possible; it is only a matter of chemistry and the right combination and interaction. We can be whatever we want —the important thing is the recipe that tells us how to mix different ingredients and what proportion. All that is required is the availability of the correct elements and tools.

Rarely does the right alchemy happen by accident. It requires discipline of the mind. Discipline means observing our mind and analyzing the nature, orbit, impact, and effect of every thought. The mind has the ability to release and process thoughts that, from tiny seeds, grow into waves of vibrations that result in actions and a manifested reality.

A clear mind can perceive reality. In fact, it defines as real only what it is accustomed to perceiving, thinking, and seeing as possible and acceptable. Everything you can imagine is a potential reality. Observing the mind is like trying to locate ourselves in a house of mirrors; what we see could be us, or it could just be the reflection of what we think we are. The mind thinks, feels, and reacts to what it perceives based on a binary system of polarity. The task of the mind is not to decide but to compare and process.

As human beings, we are not the minds; we are not what we think or feel. Rather we are spirit blown into a human body by the Primal Creative Energy. With its thoughts and feelings, the mind is a tool that serves the purpose of our soul. Consciousness must direct the mental processes that, without guidance and supervision, would be a massive, untamed powerdriven by the need for control, approval, and the countless desires of the ego. The ego that is by nature instinctive, protective, reactive, and separate can dramatically restrain the vastness of the mind and, at the same time, can enhance its power, connection, progression, and creation. The brain can accept, work, and develop only what thinks possible.

Discipline helps us expand our belief systems and explore new neural pathways suitable to perceiving and accepting reality. These actions make us free human beings, able to understand, project and create without limits.

The Crystallization of the Self

Discipline is based on the practical concept that projection creates reality. What we are, feel, and desire takes on the form of an intention internally and manifests externally as a projection. This projection impacts the circumstances of space and time, drenching them in our essence. It is an offshoot of ourselves, pregnant with the intent of our psyche. Our projection can affect the present environment and the near future, creating the conditions for it to manifest and prosper. The proportion and precision with which this happens are determined by the coherence between our deep intention and outward projection, the contents of our subconscious and the will of the conscious mind, and between what we fear to be and what we are. Reality, therefore, faithfully reflects our projection, showing us facets that need changing, situations that need to be processed, and facts that need to be accepted.

Knowing ourselves is the purpose and beginning of real life. Otherwise, we fashion our reality based on a false image of ourselves and create an environment that does not serve our true intention. Our reality, known and accepted, is the base from which to relate, perceive, process, and act. To grasp the reality of a given situation, we have to face it and experience it from our reality first. It is correct to say that our journey results from the projection of our consciousness and the experience of our relationship with our Self. There does not seem to be much else other than this. Everything else exists because we allow it to, creating it moment by moment. If we do not have contact with our reality, the sensitivity to perceive and accept each situation, and the desire to be in the experience, life will not be real. Existence risks becoming a tangled mess made up of circumstances and decisions based on emotions, impulses, and momentary reactions that separate us from our true Self and the chance to decide our destination.

Today we are assailed by motivators to help us create success and improve our relationships, performance, and revenue. These methods intervene at the stage of conception with efficiencies and positive thinking. Many are interesting tools, but they lack the ability to remove the obstacles that prevent us from having a clear perception of ourselves and the world around us.

Any approach that does not work with neutrality on our perception of reality build a new belief system that prevents further development of truthful perception itself. The concepts that will manifest will result from the contact with the non-real. It is not consistent with the Creator's essence and nor will it serve as it was meant to. The mind's ability and its projection will create something. Still, without a clear and constant perception, the direction it takes is based on an erroneous map. The decisions will be based on facts and circumstances that are not true, and the intention will be based on coordinates that are not consistent with our authenticity and originality. We certainly can live without a clear perception, and we can still produce progress–struggling and fighting. It is what we have been doing until now. Without a clear perception of reality, we ignore the consequences of what we create with our intention, words, and actions. Our crisis is not only economic or ethical, digital or religious, but perceptive at its core. We are facing a crisis of identity.

We are disciplined, at different levels, with varying motivation and degrees of commitment. Teachers devote time and space to transferring consciousness while being impersonally personal; saints control their minds to be non-reactive; and clergy can serve without attachment. It is also true that thieves and criminals have a steely discipline in studying, planning, acting and succeeding. Terrorists have a perfect unsuspected discipline, until the moment they act. Addicts have a focused discipline in their daily search for drugs. Corrupt politicians are perfectionists at making up the most believable lies. Even lazy people discipline themselves not to work. Therefore, everyone has discipline on some level, albeit some in the paradox of unruly discipline.

The most important thing to be aware of is understanding the amount of discipline needed to stay in our current mental and behavioral orientation. Awareness will confirm the quality of our discipline and the object on which to focus it. Once we discover we are disciples, dedicated to learning and following a consistent and coherent direction, the correct question to ask ourselves is: "Disciple of what, of whom, to what degree, and why am I serving?" Serving, yes. Toward what and who are our energies serving?

Whatever manifests does so at the expense of something else. How do we then decide what to sacrifice and what to sustain? How do we choose what to take and what to leave behind? The dilemma is either "solved" impulsively and emotionally or intellectually and rationally. We can hear our instincts, emotions, and rational analysis, but our awareness needs to evaluate everything, honoring our true Self. We must make each decision serve our essence, its expression, manifestation, and evolution. Everything is expendable, except our true nature.

Our subconscious's contents and processes are the engines that drive us to react to circumstances and life, bypassing the conscious level. Our subconscious, which results from traumatic experiences, unpleasant memories, unfulfilled desires, and unexpressed emotions, shapes our personality to serve habits and fears stored in this hidden yet very active corner of our mind. Instead of believing in ourselves, we allow a thought —often the result of insecurity, fear, imagination and memories — to hypnotize us subtly like a spell. If we contemplate and discipline ourselves, we recognize these dynamics and can decide who and what to serve, what to honor and what to deliver.

When the Self is crystallized, it expresses and expands into three major phases: To be the Self, to be without Self, and to magnify the Self. *To be the Self*, we need to perceive our true essence, intuitively. This happens only when discrimination lies dormant, the subconscious is muted, and mental silence prevails. Then we realize the connection to our identity. Once we have acquired the role that identity brings with it, and once we have decided to honor it, the dedication and passion that grows in us transforms our purpose into a path of pure service. Aware that we are the only ones doing what we are destined to do, with originality and irreplaceable accuracy, we live for this, dedicating our Self to the sole purpose we have chosen. Once we have found the Self, we give it to serve others and to deliver ourselves.

Being without the Self describes a state of evolution in which action, or even an entire life, is devoted to letting our energy and abilities flow as service. Service is the most ancient, wise, and practical way to clean the subconscious and be free from subordination to the ego's folly. At this stage, the only priority is action, leaving out any other activity that is not consistent with the path.

Being without attachment to what we might lose in terms of comfort and satisfaction is to dedicate our lives to our goal. Giving one's Self strengthens and makes the Self vibrant. It makes it unidirectional yet perfectly sensitive, unintentional yet open to all, unique yet universal, experienced yet humble. Whether this crystallization takes place in engrossment, between four walls, performing a public service, in an anonymous and distant mission, or in the depths of one's meditation, is not important.

Being selfless is putting the Self into action—the individual acts out his exact nature and potential. Not talking about it or promoting it but acting it out. Besides, it does not matter if the action lives only in awareness or in an authentic experience. Under this crystallization, the discovered self increases its magnitude, and we have already taken a step towards majesty.

Now, *the Self is magnified* and expanded. This process is perceptible and irrefutable by anyone sentient and alive. The real expansion is when our spirit's vibrational frequency, direct and undisturbed, radiates through space and time to affect and transform before we even reach the people, the place, or the situation. Our Self is unquestioned and accepted — not because of an artificial status, but for the reality of our presence. We need our reputation, not to satisfy us, but to deliver our true Self.

When we are contained within the Self, any insecurity disappears. A mental and conscious context opens up where intolerance and reactivity have no reason to exist. Realization, calm, and peace are the characteristics of this state of finding and being in the Self. It is the space from which to relate, change, and evolve. In every situation, we should always be able to find ourselves within the Self. The Self is the reality in which to live, from which we make sense of what has no sense. In the methodological progression of the Self, this is the place to start.

Stable in ourselves, we gain a certain frequency that amplifies our perceptive and intuitive abilities. The coherence and consistency in being and acting evoke the ability to attract resources, contexts, and information that resonate and serve our essence. These two conditions allow us to claim our unique and original role in this life, in the space we occupy in the world. Dwelling in our Self filters through and highlights our purpose. First, we perceive the Self, then we recognize how and why to act, and finally, we are ready to do so—first perception, then conception.

The Art of Consistency

The irrepressible need to create, to keep ourselves alive, and to leave our imprint on the world around us has to be preceded and inspired by a delicate phase – perception. Without perception, there can be no conception. Without understanding the true meaning of reality, we cannot be real and consistent with ourselves, and therefore we cannot be successful. If we do not deliver our best and serve people and situations in need, we allow depression to overcome us. This is the essence of misery, suffering, and frustration.

The human being who rises above challenging circumstances exists beyond space and time and becomes free. He creates the circumstances for his and other people's prosperity and happiness. However, if the circumstances define and limit us, our world becomes small, and our actions are predictable, boring, and ordinary.

If we dare to serve our higher consciousness, instead of time or circumstance, we will experience what we do not yet know about ourselves, and we will be amazed by it. We will not wait for the right situation to be happy but will express joy even when dealing with the most unfortunate environments. We will create new and profitable conditions that will result in events drenched in our positive intention. While we all desire this outcome, there is no example in humankind's history where this has happened without a life of dedicated discipline.

The consequences of an unconscious use of the mind, and therefore being a victim of our mind, are evident if we look at our lives' progression. We find that we go from one misleading thought to another, even if this drives us to act in a diametrically opposite way of our true Self. Therefore, we must first perceive reality as it truly is and then conceive a consistent, disciplined progression. We need to use our minds to serve our souls. From the teachings, we know that we must understand the pros and cons' fluctuation and then live along the diagonal between the soul and reality.

Life is not static but in constant evolution and transformation, and our discipline must always be adjusted accordingly. For this reason, discipline must be both strict and flexible. The problem lies in understanding when to be one or the other. To find out, we need to know why we are applying discipline into our lives.

Phylogeny is the study of life, from the first single-cell molecule to modern man. This science recounts evolutionary change, from the first forms of life in the aquatic environment to the transformative path that led us to finally become human, in an extraordinary adventure in which life, stronger than anything else, has shown its excellence. Ontogeny, the science that studies the individual's growth from conception to death, found that human beings trace nearly the same progression in their biological evolution. They move from gestation in the amniotic fluid, as rich in salt as a miniature ocean, to embryonic life, to life after birth of breathing, rolling, crawling, and walking. Challenges and changes are the same, constant and inevitable. Organic life, equipped with intelligence and energy, found a way to prevail, continuing to adapt and improve, surviving disasters of all kinds. With its own consciousness, organic human life came to terms with free will and decision-making, strongly affecting our physiology and psychology.

In the history of phylogeny, all along this amazing journey, life has never ceased to be faithful and consistent to its core, the nucleus that keeps it alive. The discipline of life has led itself to grow and express in spite of everything – flexible in understanding when and where to be used, and strict in being ready to sacrifice anything, except the essence of itself.

The stages of evolution are the journey along which we acquire wisdom about life, ourselves, and our relationships. In every area, we move from mere apprenticeship to mastery as we and our discipline evolve to fit each stage. Where are we then in our human, mental, professional, and relational growth? Are we novices, apprentices, practitioners, experts, or teachers? In this context, "where" is not a place, but the situations in which discipline can run aground – in which we find obstacles that impede progress and raise doubts about the effectiveness and coherence of what we are doing. Through self-observation at each stage, we investigate what is and is not working and what is and is not flowing to discover what prevents us from successfully relating to something. Through that observation, we can understand the phase of life in which we find ourselves. Honest observation and evaluation highlight the dysfunctionality of the moment, so that we can resolve it in a timely manner, bringing out the critical priorities in each situation through the application of our discipline.

We can define it as dysfunctional, any state, trend, or process that disrupts or impairs our mental and physical balance or our sense of freedom. Balance and freedom are the qualities that allow us to be ourselves and express ourselves successfully. They enable human beings to expand and transform without changing essence or purpose. Perceiving our sense of balance and freedom, we can diagnose the blocks that prevent our evolution from learning where to focus our discipline. It can also provide us with an accurate image of our discipline's quality and quantity in specific areas: objective and practical, temporal and transformative, mental and unconscious, behavioral and vibrational. These aspects consist of the circumstances of the moment, the cycles and stages of life and the different states of our evolution.

A circumstance is an objective condition that helps determine a situation including logistics, lifestyle, habits, and relationships. Certain circumstances repeat over time. We base our lives on conditions with the most suitable polarities to facilitate our objective – how to be ourselves. We can be subject to circumstances or escape them and, at the same time, influence them. We can help create them with unconscious actions or induce them consciously. We need discipline to overcome them, while at the same time, they are the reason that we are not disciplined. Often, we bend or surrender to the circumstance. It does not matter whether it is distracting, exciting, or scary — what matters is how we can use all circumstances to continue evolving, staying true to ourselves and our purpose.

Our subconscious's contents mainly determine our attitude toward the circumstance, creating such a strong influence that, despite our conscious disapproval, the subconscious maintains the unpleasant circumstance. This dissonance depends on our level of denial and our joy or fear in facing life. It happens all the time, at every level, be it personal, social, or in the work environment. Science confirms that processes taking place in our subconscious mind trigger our physiological and mental dysfunction, including disease. Dysfunctions express themselves as certain syndromes. That is why, by clearing the subconscious and addressing the circumstances, we can release the subconscious load, our psychic toxicity, and finally change our circumstances.

In any case, discipline needs a purpose, and it needs to follow a path from the point of the adverse circumstance in which we find ourselves to a more desirable one. This is the power of projection. It traces an energetic bridge between our arrival point and us that will create the reality necessary for us to reach it. Our intention rises above the given circumstances and projects forward. Intention is essential. Despite the circumstances and whether we recognize our true essence, it provides a strong desire to elevate ourselves beyond the life cycles, evolution stages and our subconscious' contents.

The cycles and stages of life are the changes and transformations in the existence of each human being. An essential aspect of human beings is their intuitive ability to understand who they are and project it into the future with applied intelligence in order to have an appropriate strategy. We require awareness to take us with grace and consistency to where we want to go and need the energy to move physically and mentally from who we are now to who we want to be. Awareness, intelligence, and energy, each with its cycle and growth process, need to maintain certain relations so that the expansion along the mental and spiritual path is balanced and we can be successful. The rhythms of the cycles and their proportions are crucial for freedom. Each stage has different needs, stimuli, and interests, and for each phase, we must reinforce and recalibrate our discipline.

The Process of Thought

Something interferes with the process of being honest and acting in harmony with the natural evolution of success. To understand what is affecting the simple innocence of being ourselves, requires that we know where we are resisting our expression, what motivates us to act, and how to apply self-discipline. In this understanding, we need to study the anatomy, physiology, and psychology of the creative process of thought and, at the same time, its subconscious counterpart.

The responsibility for the quality and flow of thoughts is our own; therefore, we have no chance of discovering our reality unless we discipline ourselves. Ultimately, everything is a thought, and how we process each thought is our life. A thought can depress us, elevate us, heal us, or make us sick. The mood, feeling, and desire that a single thought brings can lead us to happiness or chemically turn our own body against us.

What would happen if we could trust what we think, knowing it is consistent with our profound nature, knowing it is an accurate reading of our reality? When we discipline ourselves to observe the mind, consciously supervising the intellectual process, we gradually come to understand the dynamics and stages between the seed of a thought and its resulting action and distill the quality of each step in the process of creation and manifestation. Every thought must confirm our highest vision, free us, elevate us, expand us, and have an equally inspiring impact on others. Its positive impact has to be contagious. Instead of continuing to perpetuate and show our worst side, instead dare to manifest our best side.

Paradoxically, the burden of responsibility caused by a righteous and conscious action, nurtured in a clear and forward-looking mind, often feels heavier than the burden of its opposite. Revealing our best, we establish a scenario, an attitude and a magnitude that we will then have to honor. Thoughts and actions nurtured by emotions are victims of prejudice and, when filtered through past experiences and perceived dreadful consequences, are misunderstood. These dynamics are subconscious and hidden, and, despite good intentions, they can prevail because of a momentary loss of awareness. When this happens, we do not realize it. We recognize it only when it has already happened, and it is like waking up from a dream without knowing when and how it started. Guided by a hidden authority, it continues to occur without us being aware of it.

Constant observation helps us understand when this is happening and allow us to decide whether to avoid it or not. To prevent this hidden authority from slipping into our perceptive and creative mental processes and making critical choices for us, we need a habit of constant discipline. Here is the need to be present and aware of what is happening at the very moment it happens. This is the most concrete and excellent form of meditation. *Being in the moment* — this is the goal we strive for and the state where realization dwells. If we consider what *being in the moment* implies, the essence and the potential of being here and now becomes apparent.

Thought is a perfect microcosm, a seed, complete in itself and with its own intention. Once released, has its own destiny. The mind performs its projective function through its thoughts. Thought is animated by its essence, supported by its structure, given a specific vibrational frequency and radiance, and released at a crucial longitude and latitude. Thought manifestation requires discipline to maintain its characteristics and essence. Thought is a powerful reality projected in space and time.

The subconscious mind can distort the true nature and completeness of a thought if it clashes with the usual mental patterns and simply does not feel familiar. A thought is pure energy; preconceptions can alter it, but it never dies. It cannot be destroyed. It can be processed, elevated or degraded.

The teachings show us that the intellect uses three basic lenses to process a thought: the negative functional mind, the positive functional mind, and the neutral functional mind. Respectively, these approaches are protective, projective, and meditative. These functional minds manage our thinking. Ideally, it follows a three-step process. First, each thought passes through the scrutiny of the negative mind, the fastest of the three minds, to recognize every possibility of danger, in order to protect ourselves. Next, the positive mind highlights and expands the strengths that favor success and clarifies whether it is worth the risk. However, if the negative mind finds the positive mind to be weak, it hypnotizes it, causing it to search for memories that support the subconscious negative opinion. Finally, the neutral mind observes the negative and positive assessments to grasp, with the accuracy of intuition, the reality of what actually is. Then in awareness with intelligence, we act.

Any thought not processed through the three functional minds, especially if it bound with strong emotions, ends up in the subconscious. It will exist in us as if a ghost trapped in a house. It may seem forgotten, but it will continue to affect our decision-making capacity, our ability to attract, indeed, our whole reality. Eventually, we will decide; eventually, we will act either in our favor or to our disadvantage. In this way, the thoughts in the subconscious become our patterns and habits. When translated into action, they will use the customary neural networks, the usual routes that will lead to a predictable result.

Through our discipline, we can decide which thought to identify with and ride a wave because it is consistent with our true nature. If the thought honors our essence, we process it through the mental functions to be further through facets and projections. Therefore, it is not important if we have the most brilliant thought or idea, but the way we allow ourselves to accept it and process it will confirm it or not. We can be the master creator, the unwitting slayer, or the helpless hostage of each thought.

Thought is an energetic entity, as is the human being. Man has a spirit that animates him, a structure that supports him and allows his journey through space and time, with his strengths and weaknesses and with an innate capacity for expansion or contraction. He emits a unique and original vibrational frequency, and he emanates light in proportion to what he vibrates. He has precise coordinates from which to begin his journey in life and a distinct course continuing it. Man is all this, together with the innate ability to deliver himself and come to his destiny or fate.

We must know our infinite nature – our paradoxes, our virtues and flaws, skills and challenges, ambitions and intolerances, orbit and destination. In this finite world, we are born with our infinite nature unknown to us. Our job here is to explore our unknown while we live the game of life. We live through joys and sorrows because, through the extremes, we are confronted with what we do not know about ourselves in order to discover it. Behind every limit – fear, inadequacy, taboo, or preconception – lies the transcendent ability to experience our unknown and understand who we are. Just as a thought can be veiled and compromised by our belief systems – what we believe is right or wrong, what we are willing to accept or refuse – in the same way the subconscious dynamics can corrupt the Self. Like a thought, the human being impacts on the environment, others and himself, with resulting consequences. It is necessary to observe each of these facets, the impact and effects, and see how we feel towards them. We can only know ourselves by experiencing those trends that transform a thought or lead us to barter ourselves.

How then can we be happy, until we reveal ourselves and set ourselves free? Contemplating a thought's proliferation from a frequency wave to a concrete fact, we let consciousness test our intentions, words, and actions. From the appearance of human beings on earth to the present day, correcting our inconsistencies has always been the most extensive human challenge. People often describe indulging in confusion as a tendency stronger than themselves, and in fact, this can be true. The root of inconsistency is self-sabotage and sometimes it is stronger than the individuals are themselves. This sabotage happens within an operations center, invisible — yet perceptible — to the saboteur's eyes. It prevails over everything, sneaks into everything, sometimes convinces us of untruths, and causes us to persevere in failure. We may live an entire life led by the saboteur, loyal to it rather than to ourselves. That is why we need discipline – a discipline stronger than our habitual selves do.

Our actions, what we do, say, and intend, determine everything for us — our very lives and relationships. There is a world around us created by our actions, words, and will applied to an idea. The process of identifying with a thought, the words that follow, and the resultant actions taken are the most powerful creative form that exists - from pure energy to sound, to form and reality.

Kundalini Yoga, which uses sound current and mantras from the Sikh tradition, has a main mantra that describes the universe's creative aspect: *Ek Ong Kaar*. The progression of intention, word, and action is embodied in the mantra *Ek Ong Kaar*. In it, perceptive and creative abilities coexist. Intention is a potential condensed into a single point – *Ek*. Its size, proportion, and characteristics give it a shape, a vibration, in a word – *Ong*. Sound frequency, rich in intent, is embedded in a magnetic field that, passing through the ether, impacts the manifest, dramatizing into action – *Kaar*.

Ek Ong Kaar translates as "The Creator of all is One," or the "Creation is created by the Creator," or "I, creature, an integral part of creation, have the same matrix as the Creator." From the nondual, One, *Ek*, emanates duality and polarity, *Ong*, and the manifestation takes form in *Kaar*. It is the nature of who we are, where we come from, and where we are going.

THE VIRTUE OF NON-REACTION

There are two polarities in each one of us. One part strongly identifies with space and time, the body's boundaries and our mental patterns' narrowness. It is an ego-oriented identity, impulsive and reactive, that instinctively seeks immediate solutions and merely survives instead of consciously living. It is our animal nature. The other part of us is free from constraints, intuitive, and farsighted. It is not bothered by the immediate future but acts to facilitate the future it wants to build. It has a more expansive vision and recognizes the body and the world it inhabits, as a wonderful chance to have an experience. It does not identify with circumstances and feelings, yet it lives them intensely. It identifies with a body that is born and dies and a spirit that evolves in a constant experience of reality. These two polarities coexist in one essence, with awareness moving between them to bring balance, smooth out the rough edges, and facilitate and sometimes transcend for the Infinite Self to prevail.

The state of wonder that can occur in every single moment is indescribable. What happens when we are present is no longer an external phenomenon that happens with us or without us, but it is happening to us. Living the experience of what is happening to us is proportional to our ability to allow it and contain it. Instead of resisting, preventing, or combatting, we allow the present to unfold, and we process, in real-time, all that is happening. Therefore, *containing the experience* is to participate fully without reacting to what we feel. We are not controlling, judging, or commenting on the events, but accepting own inner process's pure experience.

Less than this, and life is not really lived, but instead endured unconsciously. The stress of trying to avoid or resist the experience leaves all the subconscious consequences of its impact and effect. Through our presence, we participate and concurrently process what is happening to us, preventing our thoughts and feelings from falling into the subconscious. Only by being in the present moment can we know the reality of the situation, person, or event to which we relate, and perceive the dynamics that evoke feelings and reactive patterns in us.

By experiencing the reality that happens to us, we discover the reality of ourselves. We see what makes us consistent with ourselves, and what complicates and contrasts within our personality. Just by being neutrally in the moment and containing the experience, there is the possibility that the circumstance may change simply because we, the observers, do not react.

To have the experience of living in the present moment, we must be silent and empty. If we have the memory or imagination of another experience, we cannot hear and perceive what is happening now. We must empty ourselves and allow this new experience to fill us up. To keep allowing it, inner silence must be constant. From moment to moment, we must renew our existence in the present, without indulging in inner-dialogue on the experience we have just had and without tensing in anticipation of what will come. If we can sustain this awareness, then there is no filling of inner space, and we can perceive what is really happening - inside and outside. In this state of awareness, we constantly and accurately locate ourselves. Over time, from the center of awareness we observe, and ultimately, we are able to observe the observer.

From a quantum physics perspective, matter exists only when we observe it and therefore, theoretically, nothing exists without us. We allow our world to exist when we relate to it. The identity and intent of the circumstance we perceive will affect us in proportion to how we react to it. This is the crux of the matter – how we respond to what happens creates our reality. Anything else, right or wrong, profound or superficial, is not relevant. Our discipline prepares us for this – our reaction to what happens. Circumstances evolve through different polarities: accusing or neutralizing, exploiting or losing, elevating or downgrading, accepting or rejecting, until the outcome — it all depends on how we respond. Our actions will crystallize a victory or a defeat that we gain by being in the relationship.

Perception and conception are in succession and reality determines the action. Victory is being in touch with reality, inside and outside, and acting in accordance with the reality of ourselves. How often do we live and act consistently with our true selves?

The happiness we are looking for lies in how true we are to ourselves. Happiness does not depend on circumstances that foster it or events that evoke it but on our ability to handle situations even under the most adverse conditions. Being in the present moment does not mean stopping time. It means to be in tune with it, synchronizing our clock of reality, finding the rhythm of time, the frequency to tune in to reality. Being in the right place at the right time means recognizing that what is happening is happening to us now. Everything happens and will keep happening with us or without us. If we miss what is happening to us now, we miss our own life. If we miss what is happening, we miss the opportunity to be happy.

We spend our life speculating on what might happen, or brooding over the past with regret, avoiding the reality of the moment that is far richer and more difficult to contain. Living the present moment is exciting, transcendent, and enlightening, because it is what it is. Not being in the moment is as if, on the stage of life, we point the lights where the action happened before or where it will happen next, while the current action is happening with our attention in the darkness. The way we interact with our experience in real time will build the future, delivering it into the hands of our destiny or our fate. In this play we are the protagonist, the antagonist, and the lighting technicians. We are the subject, the object, and the awareness. We are the observed, the observer, and the one who observes the observer.

How can we nullify our internal saboteur that pushes us to maintain life as it is, not knowing ourselves or being able to express ourselves, not believing in what we feel, and, ultimately, understanding what is true and what is false? The answer is discipline. Our inner work leads us to the highest end that discipline can achieve, the place where we experience being free. Each of us has something in particular, faceted and packaged according to how we have processed and digested our experiences. That something prevents us from relating to situations, people, things, or ourselves directly, neutrally, and in real-time. Understanding the nature of this block contains not only the solution, but also the potential mission of our entire lifetime.

We react to something with feelings of repulsion or attraction, pain or pleasure, interest or indifference. Our subconscious memory contrasts these sensations and influences how we manage them while distorting what we are feeling. What we are feeling becomes our inner discussion between the conscious and subconscious. Subconsciously reacting to what we feel will inevitably lead us back into our usual patterns, taking us away from the awareness of what is actually happening.

We have already seen that we can educate our minds to perceive clearly, which is fundamental, indeed imperative. However, how many times in life do we grasp what is right and then end up in the wrong? How often is our perception correct and in reacting to what we feel, be it anger, happiness, frustration, or something else, we lose the ability to communicate clearly, understand, negotiate, resolve, or simply accept?

Our life needs to be uncluttered and clean. We cannot accommodate reality, or create it, by forcing it into old and inadequate schemes. The light of awareness must be flexible, able to focus or expand as needed, and illuminate dark corners. Freedom is recognizing and accepting reality, projection is co-creating it, attention is containing it, intention is connecting to it, and happiness is to appreciate with gratitude whatever real thing manifests.

Reacting is ignorance and denial. Our real Self lay under those mechanisms that induce reaction. In this life, there is no reason not to be happy, radiant, and healthy except for our subconscious content, which consists of crucial limitations to cross, fears to exorcise, memories to let go of, thoughts to process, and psychic toxicity to drain. The subconscious is the watchdog of the Self – it performs its task by obstructing the Self's innate ability to relate to itself and the rest of the universe. The subconscious gives rise to duality, and it is the only obstacle to feeling perfect, undivided, and complete.

In the Sikh teachings, there is no duality: "True in the beginning, true through the ages, You are true now and always will be." True and perfect before, now, and after - forever. What lies beyond the Infinite Self? Nothing.

Life is the distance we must cover to achieve our destiny. The universe is our playground, and death is a new cycle of the same perpetual existence – it is like the night before the day returns. No experience is good or bad, just distinct. Consider for a moment, knowing who you are and being aware of your life's purpose. How would that feel? The completeness of the Self is strengthened by the mastery that belongs to it. The result is the achievement of a strong presence emanating the truth of ourselves, palpable with no need to explain in words or actions who we are because we are dwelling in our Self. Our purpose becomes a real mission, the reason for our life.

Presence and purpose clearly map out the diagonal path to reach our destiny. The only impediment lies in subconscious blocks and reactions that can sometimes hinder us, like a virus in a healthy body, with just one single thought. When the subconscious is congested to the point of saturation, it can release a penetrating thought into the conscious mind that soon prevails over all others and becomes so dominant that it subjugates the person. One single thought can occupy our attention, drain our energy, distract us from our purpose, mislead our nature, and weaken our will. If we look at ourselves, it is not difficult to list a handful of these thoughts that behave like cyclical torments, returning to intrude again and again. Intellectually unsolvable and immune to reason, these thoughts take precedence over entire periods of our lives. A thought like this can intimidate, hinder, or delay the natural progression of the Self. This is a potent form of self-sabotage.

Reacting to these penetrating thoughts results in stress. Rather than containing or not reacting, we choose to avoid stress by relating to something different. Often this creates additional stress that takes twice as much time and energy to recuperate from. We are trying to escape from a reality that we believe we cannot deal with, and we complicate life instead of making it easier. It is important to understand that we do not need a solution to what is happening. Instead, we must have the patience to wait, feel, and contain. Patience, the infinite kind of patience, is nothing but love.

When we react, we slam against the event with the intent of overcoming it. We try to get something, to pursue things. When patiently we contain our reaction, dwelling in stillness and awareness, we allow consistent things to come to us. Chasing after things or results, we may manage to achieve some things, but by keeping still, everything will come to us. When we stay consciously still, we open up a space in which we can accept reality. It is possible only if we remain in the creative domain of *Ek Ong Kaar*, where nothing can move us from who we are. However, even if we remain firm in containment, the experience arouses feelings, sensations, moods, and impulses. We need to act neutrally and wisely in response to circumstances and transcend these emotions with an attitude of listening and vastness.

To achieve mastery over the mind, to be successful, and to allow the flow of prosperity, it is necessary to enter into a process of attention, focus, and organization. This is possible through discipline. Mastery is not difficult or arduous. More complex and challenging is how to maintain this success. These two phases have the same relationship that exists between winning and persevering. The dynamics that complicate persevering are the result and consequence of success itself. Ancient wisdom dictates that we intuitively calculate these factors before they occur, that is, before having achieved success when intention is still dawning.

The amount of resources, relationships, and opportunities resulting from success require an incredible quality of containment and integration. Containing a situation has nothing to do with controlling it, but the exact opposite. It is the ability to resist surrendering to the urge to control what is happening, and instead exercise control over ourselves. If we can discipline our self to control the facets of our personality, instincts, and reactivity, we do not need to control anything else.

Our sense of identity, self-confidence, clarity about our intentions, and our mission's orbit and impact must be consistent with our true Self. We must practice until this understanding is routine. We must nourish it and allow its gradual and intuitive progression. The nervous system has an adaptive capacity to contain the sensory experience, without instinctively translating it into an immediate response with an unforeseen consequence.

Presented with a kind or unpleasant situation, exciting or shocking news, if we try to allow, accept, and maintain the experience that is happening to us, we discover what containment is. Containment is not something to do. It is not imploding or shriveling up. Instead, it is consciously allowing, sensing and feeling. Allowing ourselves time to accommodate the experience, we can observe our potential instinctual reactions, both conscious and unconscious.

When we transform our physical and emotional state, and perceive the immediate recurrent answers, which arise from memories of unhealed wounds, we recognize them as potential biases that attack or avoid what is happening. This is the process of distillation of the reality of the experience – it takes place by filtering, not suppressing the reactive fluctuations of our personality and the shadow of our hidden agenda. Through this process, we obtain the neutrality necessary to understand the energy that we are experiencing and the true meaning beyond the context of form and content. At the same time, we eliminate every psychic toxicity, digest and assimilate each element that promotes growth. In this way, what we need to forgive and forget does not become a subconscious burden, but, instead, is released during the experience itself.

At the same time, this dynamic influences what we call an "event" that may be a situation or a person. Because through containment and distillation we can observe and intuitively feel what causes the event, we create a change in the event. This ancient and wise approach is indispensable and relevant today. At this transition to a new age we can withstand the incredible pressure from shifts on social, mental, and energetic levels, through compassionate containment, processed through conscious understanding, and lived victoriously. "Be and let be" is the highest goal and the only way to survive as we enter the Age of Aquarius.

In these challenging times, we must confront with awareness every illness or state of imbalance. Through its neural patterns, the mind constructs the conditions of imbalance and self-sabotage. Instead of fighting the states of distress, we can decide to yield and give it the time and space required. Relaxed compliance leads to a full relationship with the discomfort and thus we can transcend it.

We progressively dissolve into Infinity, no longer identified as self, and access unlimited understanding and regeneration possibilities.

This happens when we temporarily leave the existence of doing, to lean back on the non-existence of non-doing. The first is forced and finite; the second is free and infinite. Today, any other approach to the human condition's vicissitudes cannot bring concrete, creative, and elevating effects. Beyond clarity and foresight to consciously perceive and create, we need external discipline that facilitates states of consciousness, physical vitality, and emotional adaptability.

The Age of Aquarius and the Transition we are Living in

Since the 1960s, spiritual masters from the East and the hippie movement have spoken of the coming of a new era. The Dawning of the Age of Aquarius is the title of a song from 1969. In our teachings, the earth's axis shifted on November 11, 1991, signifying the beginning of the Age of Aquarius. There was a cusp period presiding that date and similarly another cusp period adjusting to the change after that date. Meditation is most important during this change of age. Yogi Bhajan described the impact of this change on humans' psyche based on the relation between the earth's magnetic field and the human electromagnetic field.

....

The Aquarian Age is totally a reverse gear of the Piscean Age,
because love shall mean nothing but a total sacrifice. Total
sacrifice brings total understanding. Total understanding brings
total love[4]

....

[4] Yogi Bhajan, May 14, 1970

The age has changed many times before. From 4000 BC until 2000 BC, it was the Taurus era, a time of tremendous growth. From the period, we see archaeological finds of great cities and outstanding accomplishments. After that, there was the Age of Aries, from 2000 BC right until zero, an era of warriors, such as the Arians. It was the dawn of the concept of law and justice, and it is in this age that the Vedas were born in India. From the year zero to the year 2000, we have the Age of Pisces, an era marked by faith. From 2000 to 4000 is the Age of Aquarius, the era of experience. During this time, spirituality will be very strong, we will experience the Kundalini and have extrasensory experiences. Our attitude towards work will change and evolve. Different cultures are going to compare one another, and the information load is going to confuse us.

During the cusp years of the Aquarian Age, the transition to the new will be a big challenge, especially for those born in the Age of Pisces used to a certain progression of life. There will be a pervasive feeling of emptiness, and people will face significant challenges. Behaviors that were effective in the past just won't work anymore, which will create various mind disturbances.

The Magnetic Expression of the Self

The primary purpose of discipline is to enhance the frequency and magnitude of perceptual and containment skills. This authoritative and aware guidance of our own being consistent with authenticity awakens our radiance. This radiance is the expression and emanation of the human electromagnetic field that ultimately decides the quality of life's resources and destination. The magnetic field harmonizes and expands when our relationship with the Self is stable.

The subconscious contents and dynamics create alternatives to ourselves, existing as false identities and conflicting personalities that distract us from harmoniously finding our own identity. The cooperation between the authentic self with the ego and the intellect creates a personality that, far from being consistent with our identity, is a projection of how we want to appear in the eyes of others. At the same time, it has a structure that allows us to face life with less suffering and less vulnerability.

In harmony with the laws of polarity that keep the universe in balance, the existence of our personality naturally brings forth an opposite and conflicting personality, that we call the "shadow personality." These two polarities, although not always understood, are clearly recognizable. Yet, the biggest problem is that the oldest and most obscure subconscious content establishes an unknown authority that moves our life strings.

Experiences and memories that we have not processed from conception to childhood occupy the subconscious, producing belief systems and habits that generate a psyche, a "hidden identity" that obscures the authentic self. This identity driven by its needs and resentments desires revenge. The many needs and resentments are so compelling that they form a "hidden agenda." The "hidden identity" wants to follow the predictable ways it has learned in childhood, the patterns it already knows. Thus, it uses manipulation, screaming, and crying like a child. To be able to interact with others and collect what it believes is its due, it casts a "reactive personality" that manipulates environments, relationships, and events to get what it wants. It wears a "mask" in an attempt to deceive others.

So long as the relationship with the true Self does not solidify, the hidden self will dominate with its reactive personality and its complaints, and the electromagnetic field will not expand. Whatever we achieve feels empty, and life has no enjoyment. As a rule, without discipline, these factors make the personality itself feel insecure. The mask continues to protect and conceal reactive personality's intention to meet the hidden agenda's urgencies.

With discipline, we can consciously use our personality's qualities to achieve, obtain, and elevate. We can see the facets and motivations of the shadow personality that may suggest new scenarios and possibilities. We can "break" the mask to reveal the reactive personality. Then, recognized and pacified, we overcome the contents of the hidden agenda. The hidden self is the inner child crying for attention that can be calmed down with acceptance and a loving embrace. Our unexpressed strength lies in this child. We cannot fix the child; we simply need to love it.

Once we are past these blocks, the flow of energy stabilizes, balancing each element and the mental and physical systems. In the first phase, we reach the relationship with the Self, and life begins to flow in the evolution of the Self's realization. In the second phase, we sacrifice the Self's attachment and allow it to accomplish its purpose. In the third phase, we experience the magnificence of the Self.

In the first phase, the magnetic field settles on a vibrational frequency consistent with the Self's essence. Being attractive, protective, and communicative, it releases a frequency that draws resources to facilitate our path towards our destiny. In the second phase, with constant devotion, the human being's concentration aligns with its mission, reinforcing the magnetic field's frequency and originality.

In the third phase, constancy and continuity of flow in the magnetic field transform the subconscious content. The psyche remains consistent and tolerant, experiencing union with the universal psyche, causing a strong sense of belonging, awareness, and the absence of limitations. The electromagnetic field then expands and radiates in proportion to the amount of projective clarity in recognizing and being ourselves; this depends on how clean our subconscious mind is.

When the electromagnetic field is in harmony, it increases self-confidence, the ability of containment, the range of action, and the courage to explore new ways of being and expression. It creates the conditions for consistency and endurance and the caliber to dedicate ourselves to commitment. It gives us the ability to keep our word, to be nonreactive and noble. It gives charisma and graciousness.

Life is a vibration expressed by the electromagnetic field. If strong, the specific frequency emits a projection that can rearrange the surrounding electromagnetic fields, so that situations and environments begin to operate in harmony with our intention. At the same time, we relate, fully exposing ourselves to something or someone while avoiding their influence on our thoughts and emotions.

We need an effective and conscious relationship between our finite self and the Infinite Self. This is done through the magnetic field, but it cannot happen if we do not know and accept ourselves. We digest our experiences, ultimately as a means to integration. Even healthy food has parts that cannot be assimilated and produce toxins that must be eliminated. The process is similar with thoughts. Every experience has an enormous educational and evolutional importance for us. Processing it creates much of our growth and we must discard the psychic toxicity. We can decide which thoughts can prevail in our mind, just as we choose what food to eat. We can recognize a thought, its consequences and determine whether to pursue them or not. A strong sense of Self can instantly recognize what promotes and what hinders its growth, what may be challenging, painful, or even beautiful, and can lead to an evolution of the Self. This is the profound meaning of *Dharma*.

Thinking less, acting intuitively, and keeping good mental hygiene are helpful in these processes. Many things happen, relationships form, the mind generates thoughts, the past generates memories, and the future anticipates dreams. Despite all this, we must live and integrate our experience. Being free to be ourselves is a big responsibility. Limiting ourselves is acting against our own consciousness.

From Reaction to Love

Reaction and love are opposite polarities, two sides of the same coin. Reactivity is an impulse response when the human psyche unsuccessfully seeks security in material things. Only with patience does the human being realize that he is not responsible for the creation and its events. Simply stated, with love and patience, we gain reassurance, and then we can rely on the pulse of the Infinite.

As conscious beings, we can choose to be reactive and limited, or patient and vast. Expressing love requires innocence. Yet, how can we be innocent when the subconscious mind is restless and agitated? We can attempt to compensate with shrewdness and intelligence, yet the most we will achieve is a temporary benefit. Awareness, instead, is always the better solution. It will give the maximum result without reacting.

When we react, we either slam against the event to overcome it by force or we evade it altogether. In both cases, we are trying to achieve something limited by time and space. However, if we are free and aware then love naturally flows into our life. The answer to everything, to mastery over life itself, is love. Staying in the intensity of the relationship, containing and accepting sensations to uncover reality is love.

There is no middle ground. Either we live and react out of fear, or live and act out of love. Can we discipline ourselves not to live in fear and to be in love? Yes!

Although, we can misdirect our discipline to live in fear, to support fear. We support fear when we refuse to see it for what it is. Some of us employ discipline to avoid fear and organize our whole life with tools to ward off fear, avoiding even the remembrance of fear. Not facing fear, not dealing with it, requires a huge effort. We may discipline ourselves to avoid fear and fear may still be within us. This means fear dictates our intention and actions. Fear inhibits us from experiencing life to the fullest. We walk on tiptoes so as not to awaken the monster, living in disguise, a fugitive to ourselves because we fear what might happen.

We feel compelled to follow a pattern that may be cold and mechanical or hot and emotional, but not free like love. Through experience, we learn about love, devoid of the pattern of fear. It needs its own space without prejudice to diminish it. It is always an interaction – bring love to the experience without rationalization or resistance. Becoming nothing so that everything flows within and through us; this is a practical experience of the Infinite. This is true when we lovingly allow ourselves to experience ourselves. Once we have this experience, then we live it and share it to magnify it.

By applying discipline to be ourselves, we banish the subconscious authority and promote love for ourselves and others. Life is a state of awareness. Love makes awareness and continual growth. In this way, discipline frees the disciple who deeply understands, because he has lived and experienced love. Fear is a consequence of insecurity and reaction is a consequence of fear. Love is a consequence of non-reaction. If we really want to live, we must learn to love – to surrender to love.

Meditation for Rebalance

September 14, 1993

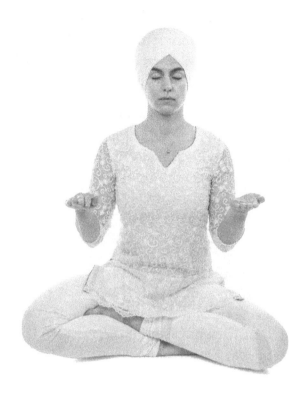

PART ONE

Time: 3 Minutes

Sit in Easy Pose with a straight spine. Bend the left elbow, hold it against the the rib cage, angle the forearm forward and upward, and bend the wrist palm face up. Raise the right arm out to side and slightly in front of the body, bend the elbow to bring the hand foreward, no bend in the wrist, palm face down. Both hands will be at the level of the Heart Center. Find a balance between the hands. The eyes are 9/10th closed, look at the Tip of the Nose and focus on the "Blue Pearl". Breathe One Minute Breath (20 seconds inhale, 20 seconds suspend, 20 seconds exhale). Immediately begin Part Two.

PART TWO

Time: 4.5 Minutes

Maintain the posture, continue the breath and begin to pump the navel independent of the breath. The shoulders will move slightly. Continue for 4.5 minutes.

To End: Inhale deep, hold the breath tight for 20 seconds. Cannon Fire exhale. Inhale deep, draw the navel in, hold for 20 seconds. Cannon Fire exhale. Inhale deep, draw the navel in and squeeze the kidney area, hold for 20 seconds. Cannon Fire exhale. Immediately begin Part Three.

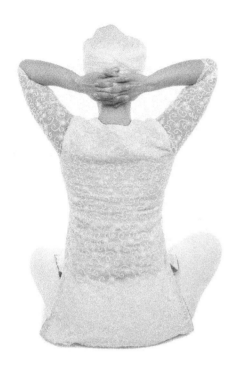

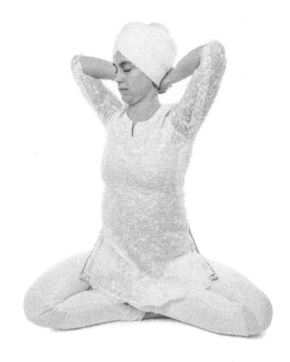

PART THREE

Time: 9 Minutes

Maintain the posture. Chant *Ang Sang Wahe Guru,* musical version by Nirinjan Kaur was played in class. **After 4.5 minutes**, inhale deep, hold the breath for 15 seconds and interlace the fingers, place them behind the neck with the elbows open wide. Exhale, maintain the posture and chant *Bountiful, Blissful, Beautiful,* by Nirinjan Kaur. Continue for 4.5 minutes.

To End: Inhale deep, hold the breath for 25 seconds as you move in the following sequence: twist to the right, hold for a couple seconds, twist to the left, hold for a couple seconds, return to center and bend forward and exhale. Inhale, repeat the sequence one more time. Relax. Stretch, shake and relax the body for 2 minutes.

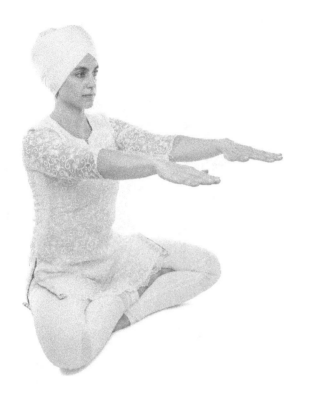
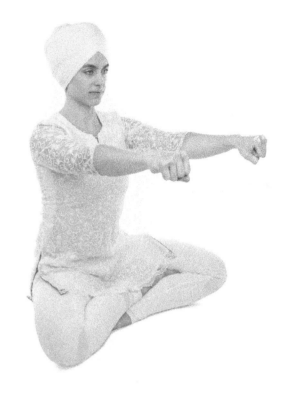

PART FOUR

Time: 10 Minutes

Remain in Easy Pose. Extend the arms straight out in front of the shoulders, parallel to the ground, left palm faces up, right palm faces down, fingers together, straight and relaxed. Eyes are open, look straight. **After 3 minutes**, begin to very slowly tighten the hands into fists and very slowly open them again. Continue this movement for 7 minutes.

To End: Inhale deep, hold the breath for 20 seconds, make tight fists and pull the navel in. Cannon Fire exhale. Repeat two more times, the third time, bow forward to Cannon Fire exhale.

Comments: As a human, you choose to act from consciousness, not from impulse. You choose to create a balance with work and relaxation.

Meditation Kriya on Haunting Thoughts

May 30, 1990

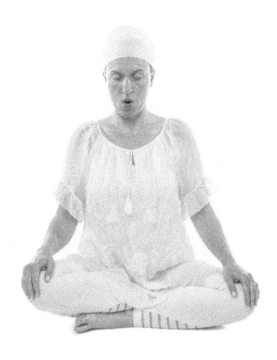

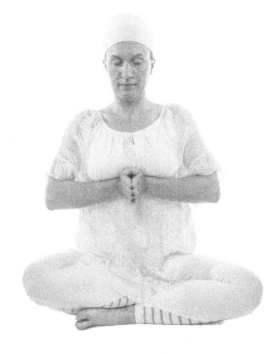

PART ONE

Time: 7 Minutes

Sit in Easy Pose with a straight spine. Relax the hands on the knees. Breathe deeply through an "O" mouth, forcefully exhaling from the diaphragm. Breath is rapid.

The inhale must be very deep and full, and exhale needs to be a powerful exhale, to have the required effect.

Immediately begin Part two.

PART TWO

Time: 17 Minutes

Remain in Easy Pose. Bring the hands together at the level of the sternum. Press the heels of the hands and forearms into the body. Press the hands and fingers firmly together, fingers point forward. Close the eyes, look at the forehead. Breathe very long and deep. Concentrate.

After 1 minute, listen to *Wahe Yantee* by Nirinjan Kaur.

To End: Inhale deeply until full and suspend the breath, sip in more air as needed to suspend for 20 seconds. Exhale slowly and consciously, control the breath as much as possible for 30 seconds. Repeat 2 more times. Relax the breath and immediately begin Part Three.

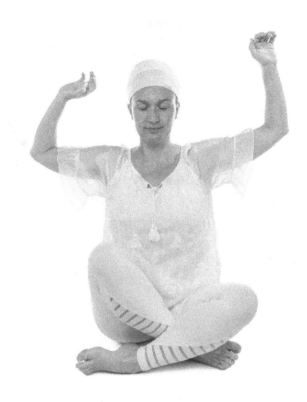

PART THREE

Time: 1 Minutes

Remain in Easy Pose. Shake the hands and arms powerfully. Simultaneously shake the legs, move them up and down. Keep the body still and only move the arms to the shoulders and the legs to the hips.

This helps to avoid joint pain in the near future.

To End: Relax.

Comments: Persistent haunting thoughts are the cause of unhappiness. They originate in your subconscious. You unknowingly follow their guidance and lose sight of your true Self and your destiny.

Meditation Kriya for Silence

November 14, 1994

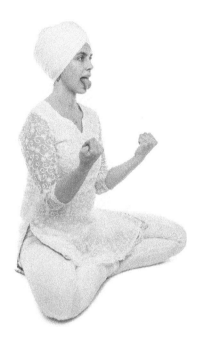 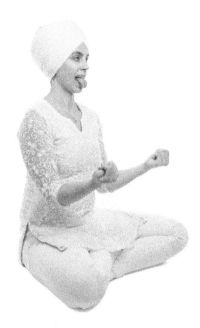 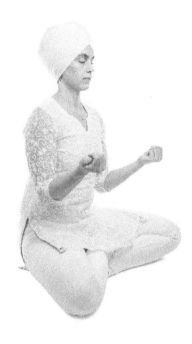

PART ONE

Time: 5 Minutes

Sit in Easy Pose with a straight spine. Place the hands in fists, palms face upward with the thumbs outside and no bend in the wrists. Bring the elbows to the sides of the body, bend the elbows with forearms forward and angled slightly up. Move the forearms quickly up a few inches and back, keep the elbows by the sides. Stick the tongue out, breathe long deep full breaths, slower than panting like a dog (Lion's Breath). Breath is slower than the arm movement. Continue for 5 minutes.

To End: Inhale deeply and tighten the entire body (fists tight, upper arms and elbows pressing the body), continue to hold the breath and twist to the right for about 10 seconds, come to center and exhale. Repeat to the left side. Inhale deep, hold for 20 seconds, tighten and try to lift the body up. Exhale and relax.

PART TWO

Time: 5 Minutes

Remain in Easy Pose. Lift and extend the elbows wider than the shoulders. Bend the elbows, lift the forearms up and out to 45 degrees, no bend in the wrists. Press the pads of the thumbs and index fingers together. Move the hands in small outward circles. Keep the spine straight and consciously put pressure on moving one arm,

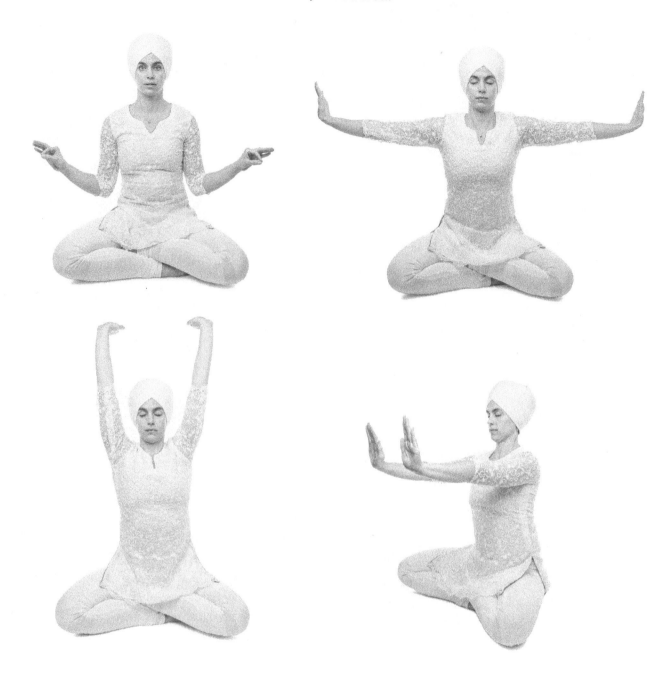

the other arm will follow, slightly turn the body. Then consciously switch pressure to the other arm turning the body. Breathe through the mouth, exhale strongly. Look straight. It is creating a magnetic circle. Continue for 5 minutes.

To End: Inhale deep, suspend the breath for 25 seconds and stretch the arms straight out to the sides, parallel to the ground, flex the wrists, palms face out, fingers point up, hold tight.

Exhale, relax. Inhale deep, suspend the breath for 25 seconds and stretch the arms straight up, elbows straight, flex the wrists, palms face up, fingers point back, hold tight. Exhale, relax. Inhale deep, suspend the breath for 25 seconds and stretch the arms straight forward from the shoulders, parallel to the ground, flex the wrists, palms face forward, fingers point up, hold tight. Exhale and relax.

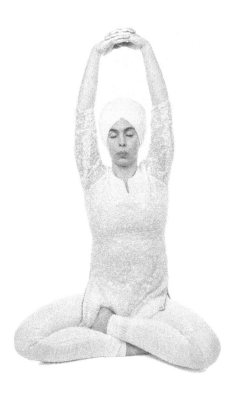
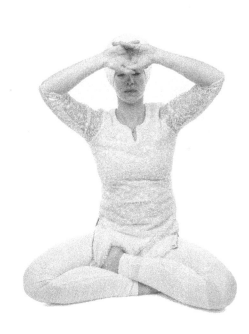

PART THREE

Time: 3 Minutes

Remain in Easy Pose. Place the fingers of one hand in between the fingers of the other hand, the fingertips do not touch the base of the fingers of the other hand, thumbs relaxed. Raise the arms straight up, elbows straight, palms face down, hold steady. Close the eyes. Whistle a national anthem. Continue for 3 minutes.

To End: Inhale deep, hold tight for 10 seconds. Exhale with a whistle and suspend the breath out for 10 seconds. Inhale with a whistle, suspend the breath for 10 seconds. Exhale with a whistle, suspend the breath out for 10 seconds. Inhale with a whistle and relax.

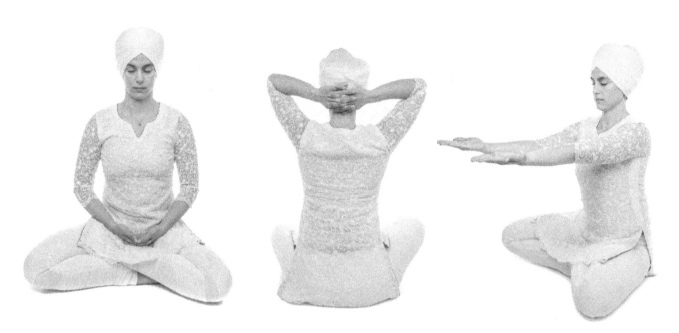

PART FOUR

Time: 11 Minutes

Remain in Easy Pose. Interlace the fingers, thumb tips touch. Place the hands in the lap palms face up and relax the breath and body. Do not move. Focus the eyes at the Tip of the Nose. Do not think, come into *Shuniya*, the state of zero. In this self hypnotic state break the attachment to the world of maya and develop your intuition. Continue for 11 minutes.

To End: Place locked hands behind the neck. Inhale, suspend the breath and twist to the right as far as possible, hold for 10 seconds. Return to center, exhale. Inhale, suspend the breath and twist to the left as far as possible hold for 10 seconds. Return to center, exhale. Inhale, suspend the breath, raise the arms forward, parallel to the ground, palms face up hold for 25 seconds. Lengthen and pull the spine up. Relax the breath, raise the arms overhead, shake the arms, legs and the whole body for one minutes.

Comments: A true sense of happiness come with the discipline of *Pratyaharaaa* bringing a neutral state, with no attachment to gain or loss and a true sense of happiness.

Meditation Kriya To Value Life

May 31, 1990

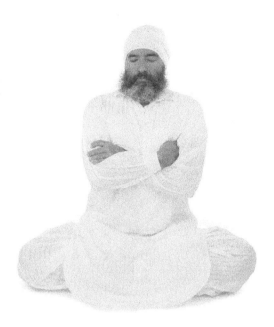

Comment: It is recommended to eat papaya with a lot of lemon before practicing this meditation kriya.

PART ONE

Time: 11 Minutes

Sit in Easy Pose with a straight spine. Cross the arms in front of the body, right arm over the left. Tuck the right hand under the left upper arm against the rib cage. Bring the left hand up and hold the upper right arm. Press the arms tightly against the rib cage, create a lock, the body will feel lifted. Squeeze the rib cage tight while pulling the arms without releasing the lock. Take a deep breath, hold it tight and perfect the posture, thereafter, breathe consciously, deep and strong. Do not relax the posture. The cheeks will become red.

After 4.5 minutes, Inhale deep, hold the breath. Wrestle between the lock and the pressure. When you can no longer hold the breath, let the breath out slowly. Inhale slowly and keep a steady slow breath. Continue for 6.5 minutes.

To End: Inhale deep, exhale, relax, shake your hands for 10 seconds. Immediately begin Part Two.

Comment: Attachment to haunting thoughts creates major insecurity. Pull as hars as possible now and release this hold.

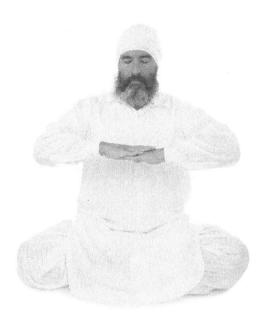

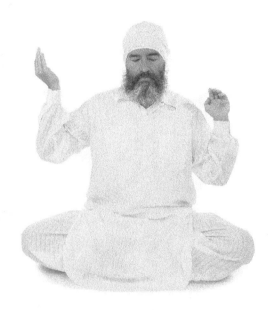

PART TWO

Time: 15 Minutes

Remain in Easy Pose. Bring the elbows out to the sides, forearms parallel to the ground, no bend in the wrists. Place the right hand on top of the left hand in front of the Heart Center. (If the left hand is dominant, place the left hand over the right.) The dominant hand presses down and the lower hand presses up, without moving the hands. Create a balance between the two forces. Breathe long, deep and consciously.

After 5 minutes, Maintain the posture and also squeeze the waistline and rib cage. Pull the belly in and squeeze the rib cage.

After 5 minutes, Maintain the posture and apply Root Lock and squeeze the buttocks.

After 2 minutes, Maintain the posture and additionally tighten the shoulders, balance the pressure between the hands for 3 more minutes.

To End: Inhale deep, hold the breath, tighten the body for 20 seconds. Exhale, relax the breath. Move the body gently, shaking the hands and rolling the shoulders for 30 seconds. Immediately begin Part Three.

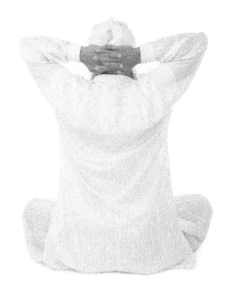

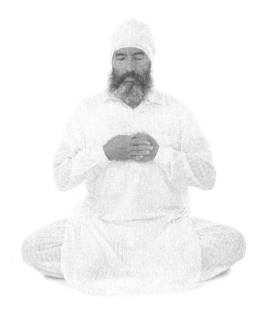

PART THREE

Time: 4 Minutes

Remain in Easy Pose. Interlace the fingers behind the neck. Push the neck backward and pull forward with the hands forcefully. The push and pull are equal and maximum to create a balanced lock. Continue for 4 minutes.

To End: Inhale deep, hold the breath for 10 seconds. Exhale. Inhale deep, inhale more, hold the breath for 20 seconds. Exhale and relax.

PART FOUR

Time: 20 Minutes

Remain in Easy Pose. Lock the hands on the Heart Center, right hand over left hand. Close the eyes and leave the body.

After 1 minute, play the gong, simultaneously with *Walking up the Mountain* by Gurudass Singh.

After 6 minutes, the gong ends. Music continues; *Walking up the Mountain* for 2 minutes, *Walk on the Cold Marble* for 6 minutes, *Flowers in the Rain* for 5 minutes, silence for 30 seconds.

To End: Inhale deep, hold the breath, circulate the breath by your mental hypnosis to every organ of your body for 30 seconds. Exhale. Inhale deep again, hold the breath, hypnotically transform it into a peaceful energy, penetrating every organ of the body for 25 seconds. Exhale. Inhale deep again, hold the breath for 30 seconds and eliminate all thoughts of the past. Exhale and relax. Shake hands for 5 seconds. Raise the arms

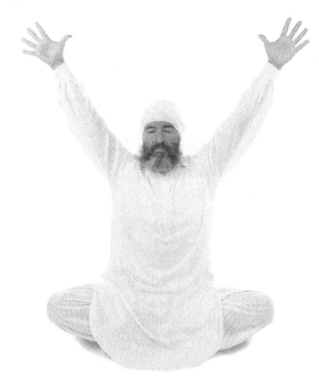

PART FIVE

up to 60 degrees, stretch the fingers wide and straight. Reach up with the hands and stretch the entire spine upward. Breathe normally for 40 seconds. Relax. Immediately begin Part Five.

Time: 30 Minutes

Remain in Easy Pose. Talk to each other and totally relax. Talk about mundane things such as what was for lunch.

Comments: When you value your own life, you also value other's lives. Pure love is the essence; self-love and love for others. There is nothing else.

Meditation Kriya Balance into Shuniya

November 3, 1994

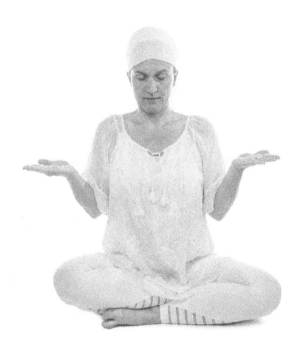

PART ONE

Time: 5 minutes

Sit in Easy pose with a straight spine. Bend the elbows and keep them relaxed by the sides. Raise the forearms up and angled slightly out. The hands are relaxed with the palms facing up. Sit calmly and quietly. Close the eyes, look at the Moon Center (the chin). Do not move. Give yourself up. Continue for 5 minutes.

Immediately begin Part Two.

PART TWO

Time: 5 Minutes

Maintain the posture. Begin One Minute Breath, 20 second inhale, 20 second suspend, 20 second exhale. Continue for 5 minutes.

Immediately begin Part Three.

PART THREE

Time: 5 minutes

Maintain the posture. Inhale through the nose, exhale through the mouth. Breathe long and deep. Continue for 5 minutes.

Immediately begin Part Four.

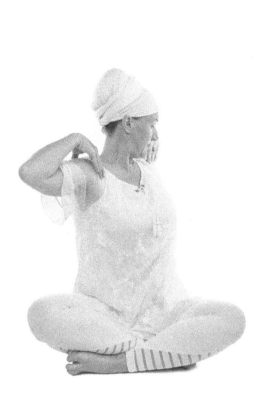

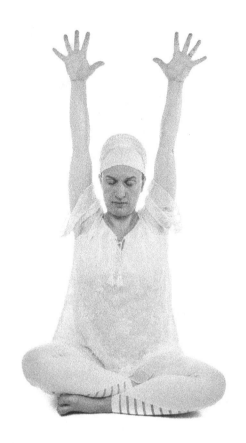

PART FOUR

Time: 10.5 Minutes

Maintain the posture. Inhale deep and totally relax into *Shuniya*, nothingness. Breathe in and out as you please, be absolutely thoughtless. Continue for 10.5 minutes.

To End: Inhale, hold the shoulders tightly. Twist left as much as possible, hold for a moment, return to center, exhale. Inhale, twist right as much as possible, hold for a moment, return to center, exhale. Inhale deep, hold the breath, raise the hands up, fingers wide and tight like steel. Stretch the spine as much as possible for 15 seconds. Exhale and relax.

Comments: In the emptiness of *shuniya*, you find fullness. Surrendering yourself, there is no longer a difference between everything and nothing. Your life becomes bountiful and complete.

Meditation Kriya to Get Rid of Haunting Thoughts

June 4, 1990

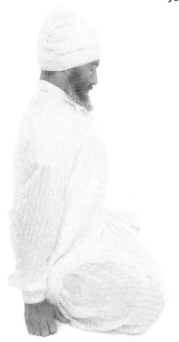

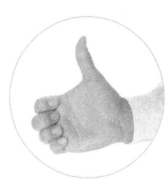

Instructions:

It is recommended to eat papaya with a lot of lemon before practicing this meditation.

PART ONE

Time: 24.5 Minutes

Sit in Easy Pose with a straight spine. Remove any rings from the fingers. Fold the fingers onto the mounds, extend the thumbs. Place the hands on the ground next to the hips, knuckles face forward. Straighten the elbows, bring the arms close to the body. Lift the chest, pull the shoulders up, apply a strong Jalandhar Bandh (neck lock), chin in toward the collarbone. Stiffen the neck like steel. Close the eyes. Breathe very slowly and very deeply. Do not lean forward.

Comments: A haunting thought may come or it may remain hidden. Either way, this exercise will release it.

After 9 minutes, maintain the posture, play *Waah Yantee Kar Yantee* by Nirinjan Kaur.

Listen for 11 minutes. Maintain the posture, continue to listen and pump the Navel Point for 4.5 more minutes.

To End: Inhale deeply, suspend the breath, pull a strong Muhl bandh (root lock) for 20 seconds. Relax. Massage the hands, move them, shake them, move the fingers, shoulders, rib cage and the neck. Stimulate the circulatory system for 1 minute. Immediately begin Part Two.

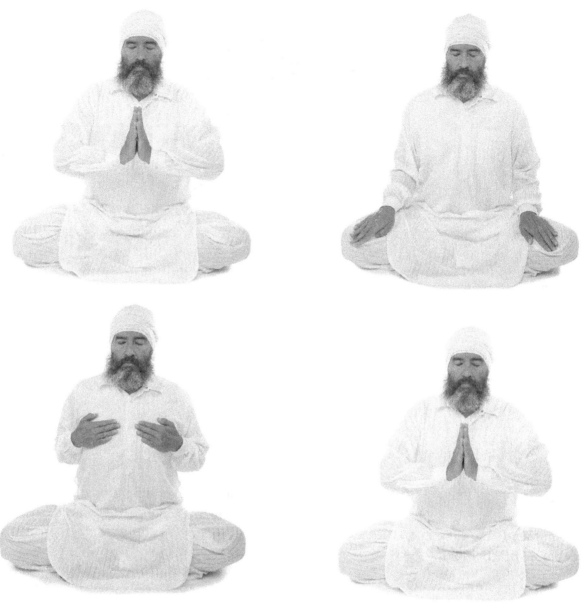

PART TWO

Time: 6 Minutes

Remain in Easy Pose with a straight spine. Repeat the following sequence:

1. Clap the hands at the Heart Center

2. Hit the inside of the knees

3. Hit the chest at the level of the heart

4. Clap the hands at the Heart Center

Continue for 6 minutes.

Comments: Make all movement strong, so that you hear the sound of the clap and the hit on the inner knee and chest. This exercise removes thoughts of grief.

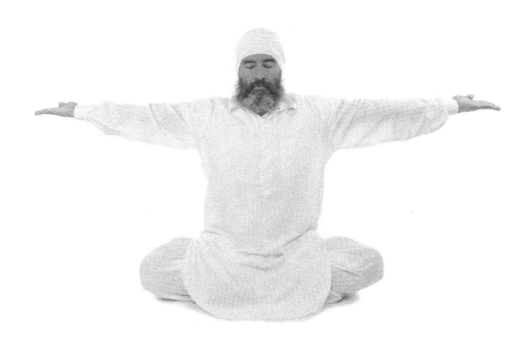

To End: Inhale deep, hold the breath for 20 seconds, stretch the arms out to the sides, parallel to the ground, elbows straight, hands flat, palms face up. Squeeze the lower back to get rid of the pain. Use the strength of the hands to squeeze the body upward. Exhale. Repeat 3 more times. Relax. Do anything light, talk to each other and relax.

Comments: Haunting thoughts are stored in your subconscious and cause you to believe and act from perceived pain, insecurities and untrue beliefs. Intuition is the solution, so that you know the cause and can see the consequences without the influence of the hidden thoughts, and stop reacting.

Meditation for Creating

September 16, 1993

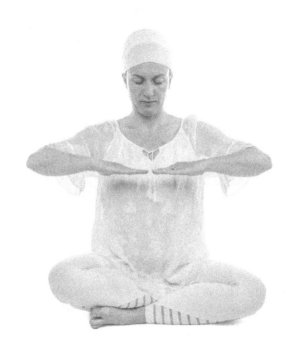

Time: 14 Minutes

Sit in Easy Pose with a straight spine. Raise the elbows up and out to the sides, forearms parallel to the ground with the hands flat in front of the Heart Center, palms face down, fingers point towards opposite hand. Saturn Fingers (middle fingers) do not touch, stay ½ inch (1 cm) apart. Focus the eyes at the Tip of the Nose, experience seeing the Blue Pearl. Breath is unspecified. Concentrate.

The forehead may become heavy as the posture adjusts. Keep your eye focus and be sure that the fingers do not touch.

After 7 minutes, Maintain the posture and eye focus. Listen to *Meditation* by Wahe Guru Kaur. Continue for 7 minutes.

Be aware of pain in your body and know that energy going there will restore the flow of energy.

To End: Music ends. Inhale deep, hold the breath for 20 seconds. Stretch the spine consciously vertebra by vertebra from the lower tailbone up to the neck. Exhale. Repeat three more times. Relax and shake the hands and body wildly. Spread the energy to all the facets of the body. Continue for 1 minute. Relax. To end the practice, move just the toes and the fingers fast, balance what has been achieved. Continue for 1.5 minutes.

Meditation to Renew Yourself to Be Simply You

September. 23, 1993

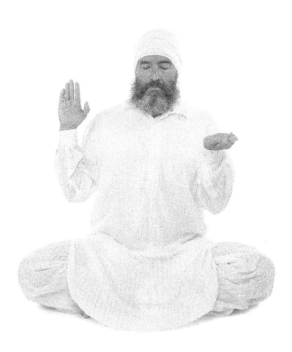

PART ONE

Time: 11 minutes

Sit in Easy Pose with a straight spine. Bend the right elbow. Raise the right hand to face level, palm faces forward, fingers straight. Bend the left elbow, keep it against the rib cage. Extend the left forearm forward, hand at the level of the heart, palm faces up, hand relaxed. Left hand is the beggar, right hand gives a blessing.

Close the eyes and go to sleep. Use self-hypnosis to get into a nap state. Do nothing, no thought, invoke a self-sleep. Listen to *Guru Ram Das Lullaby* by Snatam Kaur, softly. Continue for 11 minutes.

To End: Inhale deep, hold the breath for 20 seconds and move all the muscles impulsively, shake hard. Exhale powerfully. Repeat two more times. Relax.

Comments: Maintain your posture and sleep. Allow the mind to become pure and crystal clear and stress be relieved.

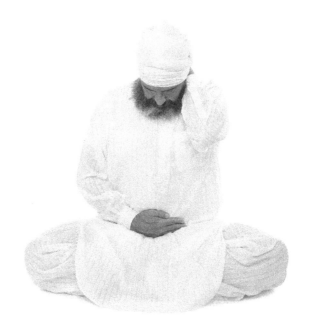

PART TWO

Time: 7 Minutes

Remain in Easy Pose with a straight spine. Wrap the left hand around back of the neck, elbow points forward, gently let the head fall forward.

Place the right hand on the Navel Point. Close the eyes. Relax the body, go into self-hypnosis.

Continue relaxing any tightness in the neck. Come into *shuniya*.

Listen to *Meditation* by Wahe Guru Kaur. Continue for 7 minutes.

To End: Inhale deeply, hold the breath for 20 seconds and press the hand at the Navel Point with maximum pressure, pull the neck with the hand with maximum pressure. Bring the entire body to a balance. Balance it with the maximum pressure the hands can exercise. Exhale. Repeat two more times. Relax and shake out your hands.

Comments: From *shuniya* comes intuition which comes from your authentic being. Happiness comes from this purity of Self. You speak, act and live from your essence, and happiness is assured.

Meditation Kriya to Mine the Mind

April 12, 1989

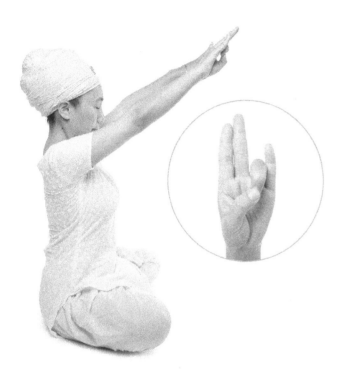

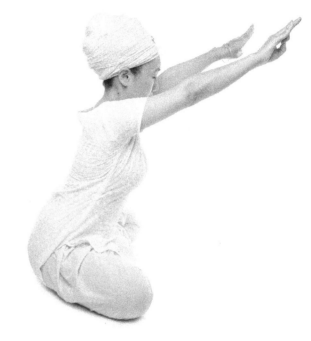

PART ONE

Time: 13 Minutes

Sit in Easy Pose with a straight spine. Place both hands in active Ravi Mudra (thumbs overlap the tips of the ring fingers, the rest of the fingers are straight). Raise the arms out from the shoulders forward and up to 60 degrees, elbows straight, palms face down. Close the eyes and concentrate on the Third Eye Point.

After 5 minutes, Play *Bountiful, Blissful* by Nirinjan Kaur.

After 3 minutes, Chant loud and clear with the music. Continue for 5 more minutes.

To End: Relax the posture. Rest in Easy Pose for 6 minutes.

PART TWO

Time: 6 Minutes

Remain in Easy Pose with a straight spine. Come into the same posture as Part One. Push the arms out from the shoulders. Close the eyes, meditate. Chant with the same music as Part One. Continue for 6 minutes.

To End: Inhale deep, hold the breath for 20 seconds and stretch forward from the lower spine, lift the arms to maintain the 60 degree angle, stretch tight like steel, bring the body into balance. Exhale. Repeat two more times. Relax.

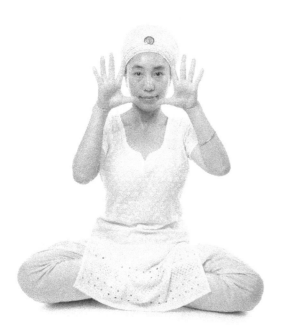
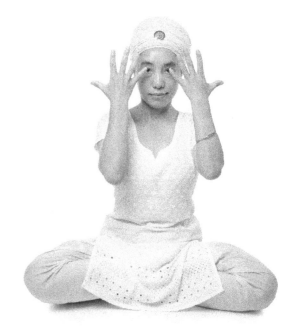

PART THREE

Time: 3 Minutes

Remain in Easy Pose with a straight spine. Bend the elbows. Place the hands in front of the face, base of the palms at the level of the chin, fingers spread wide, palms face forward. Twist the forearms and hands from the elbows, turning palms toward the face, fingers stay wide. The hand movements mirror each other. Look at the palms. Continue for 3 minutes.

To End: Relax the posture. Move the shoulders, stretch the hands, move the lower back and the entire body; move gently. Continue for 1.5 minutes.

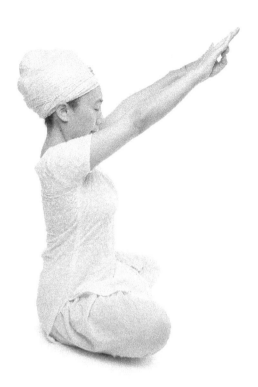
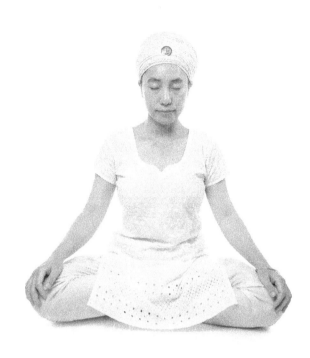

PART FOUR

Time: 8 Minutes

Remain in Easy Pose with a straight spine. Come into the same posture as Part One. Reach out strongly from the shoulders. Play *Bountiful, Blissful* by Nirinjan Kaur. Chant.

After 3 minutes, music stops, relax the posture and rest.

After 1.5 minutes, return to the posture and chant with the same music. Continue for 3.5 minutes.

To End: Inhale deep, hold tight, lock your back molars and stretch out in every way for 20 seconds. Exhale. Inhale deep, hold tight and stretch as much as possible for 15 seconds. Exhale completely. Inhale, exhale, inhale, exhale, inhale, exhale deeply, suspend the breath out, pull the navel in and stretch up for 15 seconds. Relax.

SADHANA

The Four Ashrams

Ancient Indian tradition tells us that there are four *ashrams*, or stages, in life. The first *ashram* starts at birth and continues throughout our learning phase. This is the time when we study and receive an education. The second is when we enter the world, in both job and social realms. The third is when we teach what we have learned, share the outcome of our experiences. The fourth is when we get ready to leave earthly life.

I will use my life here to explore these stages. In the first stage, I received my cultural, social, and religious education, and at the time, it seemed to me like they were the only existing truths. Now I see them as false, oppressive, or limiting truths because they lack the spiritual context needed to set one free. I studied mathematics and languages in school but what I actually learned was to be emotional, afraid and guilty. Despite the intention to give me the best education to enter society, the longer I attended school, the bigger my feelings of inadequacy became. It became harder and harder to carry this burden. As I approached the second *ashram*, my positive qualities, creative gifts, and spiritual potential occasionally surfaced. I was reluctant to show my true essence, which by now felt like a taboo. No one guided me to discover my real priorities – to acknowledge the true reality in relationships, value human qualities, understand the essence of communication, and reach for the true goal of life. Like most people, I acted out the drama between fate and destiny, an unavoidable result when upbringing lacks spiritual values and education lacks *Humanology*. When I started practicing Kundalini Yoga, my physical, mental, spiritual needs converge in a sole priority – to discover my own infinite essence and leave an imprint of this quality on the space-time planet called Earth. This is what we need to be teaching our children.

At first, in the transformation engendered by Kundalini Yoga, students find a latitude and longitude, besides the altitude from which to avoid identifying with false personalities. In ancient teachings, a spiritual name is the highest blessing one can receive from their teacher. The new name grants the student the attitude to perceive and experience their spiritual identity, their destiny. It is the matrix of the Infinite's expression within us.

The spiritual name I was given is *Sadhana Singh*, the "lion of spiritual disciplines." When I received the letter from Yogi Bhajan giving me my spiritual name, he said to meditate on it, repeat it, understand its profound meaning, and "make it work." With this new found companion, life became an exciting, adventurous exploration.

Originating from the Sanskrit root "*sadh*," which means a saintly person, *sadhana* commonly indicates spiritual practices that lead us to the realization of truth. Breaking the word into individual sounds, we find SA – infinite totality, DHA – meditation or also earth, and NA – death. Thus, *sadhana* is to die while still alive, experience the Infinite, and be a testimony of it here on Earth. To die to oneself is to let go of the insanity of the divisive ego and allow God's will to prevail and sustain us. When the interference of our limited ego is gone, we experience our unlimited spirit.

Sadhana is one of the main structures in our kundalini yogic teachings and is the basis of our spiritual life. It starts in the early morning between night's darkness and sunrise's light, between the deepest corners of the subconscious and the clearness of consciousness. I began to compile notes about *sadhana* from books, seminars, and Yogi Bhajan's words, along with my experience of *sadhana*, recording its profound meaning and its transformational experience.

Therefore, although this is not an autobiography, the author's name coincides with the title of this section. Through the practice of daily *sadhana*, we write our own biography. In the internal journey directed by our discipline, we transform the five passions into elevating instruments, and it becomes possible to distinguish the temporary from the permanent. We learn to acknowledge any action that might get us closer or further from God, avoid stirring the causes leading to unwanted consequences, not be victims of fate, and instead be the master of our destiny. What is superfluous evaporates and what emerges is our source, direction, and destination.

WHY MEDITATE?

The best starting point to answer the question "Why meditate?" is acknowledging the fact that every living being on this planet is in search of happiness. Every action and every thought arise from what we believe might lead us to happiness. We hold the belief that being happy is a birthright of all humans, except that we do not know how to achieve it. We are ready to do anything, make decisions and mistakes that compromise our future, for a few moments of happiness. By doing so, we drain *praana* from our authentic Self, ultimately resulting in unhappiness and confusion. Desperately wanting to appease our ego, we reject challenging situations that may be painful. Instead, we compensate by embracing inadequate substitutes, for a moment filling what we lack and repressing those experiences labeled as "negative" by our mind. Repressing emotional needs and desires is like swallowing a bitter bite and not digesting it or hiding the entire house's dirt under the bed and ignoring it exists. This tremendous amount of information and experiences, which we labeled as negative, does not vanish in thin air. They are stored in a vast, dark, and unknown container, which we have discussed previously, the subconscious mind.

The subconscious mind is like a hallway, quite a narrow one, between the conscious mind and the Supreme Consciousness. When this hallway is full, the communication between them becomes obstructed. The conscious mind can no longer access the help of the *akashic record*, which is the compendium of human experience, containing precious guidance relevant to our situation. The subconscious mind keeps affecting our actions and determining our personality and character.

In addition to the influences of our adult life's repressive processes, the experiences during our first eleven years shape who we are today. This period is the first cycle of intelligence[1]. During this time, events are out of our control, and repeated patterns create fears. From zero to three years old, our relationship with our mother leaves an imprint on our brain that leads to a tendency. These tendencies display as an imbalance related to the first and second chakras that manifest in our self-esteem. The tendencies established during our first three years influence us throughout our life.

From three to eleven years old, the primary influence is our relationship with our father and with the world we are beginning to discover. The child becomes consciously aware of themselves and their identity in relation to their parents. In this phase, unbalances manifest in the third and fourth chakras and relate to patience, responsibility, and discipline.

Meditation is the key to open this emotional baggage, stored and locked in the realm of instincts and habits. During the evolutional process of life, we stray further from God's will when we believe we can satisfy our need for happiness by appeasing our senses and momentary desires. The ego is supposed to give us a sense of individuality, a healthy distinction from the rest of the creatures and the creation, allowing us to live together following the rules of space and time. But when we focus our attention on the ego's needs and desires, it leads us further and further from the freedom we yearn for. We then end up creating sequences, followed by consequences, building an ego-based reality with our own hands. This is the process of *karma*, where we experience the effects of our actions.

By daily cleaning our subconscious mind through the practice of *sadhana*, we prevent the past from negatively influencing our present or future life. Meditation trains our mind to reach a superior state in which our actions and thoughts do not result in negative sequences but instead grow into the experiences we have had with sensitivity and understanding. Right action, the path of *dharma*, will not create *karma*.

1 Aquarian Teacher Level One Textbook

The Facets of the Mind

Let us briefly consider the different facets of the mind from yogic technology as presented in Kundalini Yoga technology to understand how meditation helps us purify our subconscious and free our conscious mind. We have three impersonal minds:

Buddhi – This mind perceives reality and aligns with the Infinite Identity.

Ahangkar – The ego that gives identity through attachment and emotions.

Manas – This mind controls the senses, including the subconscious mind's reactions, desires, and emotions.

In the previous Discipline section, we already discussed the three functional minds. The *Negative Mind*, the protective mind, depends on the ego and reveals the potential harm in any situation. The *Positive Mind* also is bound to ego and shows the potential in any situation. It defuses the negative mind and pushes us to act. The *Neutral Mind*, the meditative mind, is detached from the ego and stays further away, often keeping its state unknown, and thus is used less than the other two.

The drama unfolds between the negative and positive minds. Until they find their balance, they keep on running the "subconscious show." While the negative and positive minds draw their strength from the subconscious, it reinforces the behaviors we no longer want to manifest in us. These minds struggle to prevail over each other. When we engage the neutral mind, it takes only nine seconds to reach a resolution. How does the neutral mind prevail through the chaos of the other two minds? The answer is when it is trained. And the neutral mind can only be trained through meditation – that is the yogi's mind. When the balancing process is automatic and immediate, the result is that we do the right thing for the right reason. We listen. We act in compassion rather than react. We do not resist the requirements for growth. Through meditation, we clear the "dirt" from the subconscious, and the conscious mind observes without judgment and acts with wisdom.

Gurucharan Singh Khalsa explains the teaching regarding the relationship between a clear mind and prosperity in *Happiness is Your Birthright*[2],

---

[2] 1997, Khalsa Consultants, Inc.

"Prosperity, intended as the realization of one's own destiny, is the consequence which concentrically invades every level of humans. It's when the duality of the protective thought is nullified by the meditative mind, which grasps the real essence of reality. It's when the communication with our unknown is so clear and continuous that no interference might impede what needs to happen for our soul and our divinity. The ability of human beings to vibrate with the Infinite. At this point, events won't matter anymore, nor circumstances will, only the balance in this relation will."

The interaction of the three functional minds, the Negative, Positive, and Neutral minds, along with the three impersonal ones, *Manas, Ahangkar,* and *Buddhi,* create the nine aspects of the mind that display as an attitude, a position taken in relation to a situation, thought, or feeling. All nine minds are necessary, and their value is equivalent, although some might be more visible than others in individuals who ignore some aspects and highlight others. The mind evaluates these facets to choose the best attitude in a given situation.

The three functional minds are the fundamental modes of reaction each of us has. The three impersonal minds are the functions of *chitta,* the Universal Mind, and they reflect from the three *gunas,* or qualities of the original conscience. The three *gunas* are *tamas, rajas,* and *sattva. Tamas* is persistent, heavy and concealed. *Rajas* is active, creative, energetic, and the power of transformation. *Sattva* is balanced, pure, light, and neutral.[3]

By experiencing life through one's own actions and reactions, we record each step we take in the subconscious and Supreme Conscious, creating a thought pattern that prepares the mind for each new situation.

[3] Aquarian Teacher Level One Textbook

Commitment and Spiritual Growth

Sadhana is primarily food for our aura, our magnetic field. We practice in the *Amrit Vela*, the ambrosial hours before the sun rises, the time when we test our commitment to the foundation of our spiritual growth.

Sadhana is for everyone, not just for the yogis and ascetics living outside the material world. And those who aren't rich are going to find prosperity in it by attracting richness and enhancing their radiance. The outcome of a solid and consistent *sadhana* is an expanded auric body and a neutral mind capable of grasping opportunities, as well as improve the endocrine system's functioning.

Sadhana pushes us to live fully and become present. It improves our innate psychophysical abilities. When we are balanced, everything naturally flows to us. Conversely, when our aura is not strong enough, we use a protective mask. *Sadhana* gives us the chance to throw this mask away. Every day, when we sit and meditate, we clean the subconscious mind and balance our physiological systems. We take control of our minds and become the author of our destiny. No more are we victims of the whims of fate. Kundalini yoga technology teaches us that just as we eat food and drink water every day to sustain a healthy body, we do *Sadhana* to maintain a healthy mind.

According to yogic teaching, for every completed action or generated thought we create ten times more of the same thing. This means that every projection, whether good or bad, is subject to its karmic cycle of action and reaction, and the number regulating this cosmic wheel is ten. In numerology, the number ten includes everything – "everything or nothing[5]." Act, speak or think, with bad intention and ten times that negativity comes back; do it with goodness and ten times that positivity comes back. It's not a curse. It is a cosmic law. This is how Nature helps us understand, grow, and change – it is not a punishment. Thus, when we dedicate a tenth of the day to our spiritual practice, by doing two and a half hours of *sadhana*, we receive the tenfold benefit for the rest of the day. With practice, we are disciplining our minds, not running uselessly after it. In this way, we avoid suffering the effects and instead go to the center, to the cause, to become masters of ourselves.

Our self-conquest, as well as our growth, happens gradually. Every day of practice adds up, accumulating the effects of the *sadhana*. The more we practice, the more we understand the importance of discipline, as already discussed. The student, practicing constantly and honestly, can become the master. No one else can do it for you. What leads to mastery is experience. The tool is discipline, its strength is will.

Sometimes we leave our life in the hands of others, wanting to be guided and relieved of our pain. We ask mercy from God without understanding that we are God. We are overwhelmed by so much information. We abuse our bodies without understanding how much this is going to cost us in the long run. Every day of abuse takes three days to bring us back balance. Many avoid or are afraid to work on themselves. What we really are avoiding is taking responsibility to excel, to heal, and ultimately to love. Who wants to be like this when the emotional world is so fascinating? Beware. The drama of emotions with accompanying commotions and projections is a mental trick, that impedes being intelligent, aware and intuitive.

---

[5] Aquarian Teacher Level One Textbook

The Process of Sadhana and How it Progresses

The yoga process explores the union of finite with the Infinite, stimulating the sleeping energies that reactivate and balance our energetic system. The experience of becoming alchemists of our own selves leads us to knowledge through discipline and willpower. Guru Dev Singh, master of Sat Naam Rasayan, says: "Our psychophysical stability is not given by anyone, not even by God, because He is stability as He is instability, being everything."

Do you know how a sculptor works with marble? There are two ways to complete his work. The first way is to create a miniature model using an easy-to-mold material that is sent to the worksite where computers using automation in scale reproduce the model in marble. The artist never touches the material. The second way is to create a small model, prepare a sketch made of chalk in the desired dimensions, and sculpt it in the marble. The sculptor requires new tools for each piece of work for precise results. Here the artist, with their experience respects the individuality of the piece of marble, its flaws, shape, and curves. They become one with the sculpture, having obtained mastery through knowledge.

The second process is similar to *sadhana*, the first of the three fundamental and inseparable stages: *Sadhana* – the discipline; *Aradhana* – the attitude; *Prabhupati* – the mastery. In the beginning, a period of discipline is required to release old habits and instill them. The *saadhak*, one who practices *sadhana*, decides to walk the effective path of reality, not the illusory path. Standing alone facing the fear and negativity triggered by identification with emotions, the *saadhak* releases old habits. Like the sculptor, the objective is to realize one's work of art that lies inherent within the hard rock and that at times might seem unreachable. This difficult passage creates duality in the *saadhak*, divided between "old and false identity" and passing into a higher state of consciousness to reach the state of *Aradhana*.

Reaching this stage requires a huge effort and commitment for both the *saadhak* and the sculptor. Extensive tests stand in the way, such as doubt and fatigue. We must reinforce our willpower to find the motivation and the energy to go on. However, if they keep up and lock their attention on that small crevice of light that shines, proving the existence of an Infinite nature, then the mental attitude becomes consolidated. *Aradhana* cleans the subconscious, leaving room for *Prabhupati*. When we enter into this state, there is an absence of negativity, even hiding in the subconscious, because we have integrated the subconscious with the conscious mind. The individual consciousness is in communion with the Universal Consciousness for the maximum expansion of love and understanding.

A committed *sadhana* balances the brain's two hemispheres so that the central part of the brain can be functional, influencing our intuition and the entire endocrine system. This is the powerful expansiveness of the meditative mind.

The right hemisphere controls the left part of the body, expressed at the intuitive, artistic, subjective, and perceptive level, and linked to space and language. Therefore, the mantras, rhythms, and breathing in meditations relate to the right hemisphere and expand our mind; they belong to *Laya Yoga*. The left hemisphere controls the right part of the body. It processes personality, identity, the concept of time, and what is mathematical and scientifically oriented. It is rational and extroverted. *Pratyaharaa*, clearing the mind through detachment, is a function of the left hemisphere.

Yogic philosophy recognizes several stages of consciousness, referred to in kundalini yoga technology as the meditative mind. The first stage is called *jagrat* (waking), in which the mind and the sense organs work together. We recognize a sense of impression from the past and understands it in a physical sense. The next stage is *swapna* (dreaming), in which the sense organs are not awake while the mind continues to be active. The dream, created by the release of unresolved subconscious material, mimics the waking stage. In this stage, we are unable to sleep peacefully. The next stage is called *sakupath*.[6] (dreamless sleep), a deep sleep stage in which both the senses and the mind are at rest. We are unaware of any identification, thoughts, and emotions and are united with the Self. *Turiya* (sleepless sleep) is the final stage, although some scholars divide it into different levels. This stage is not experienced by the senses and not understood by the mind. We experience bliss and see the union of the finite and Infinite while remaining aware of our own consciousness (this stage is called intermediate *Samadhi*.) The next level, *Turiyatita*, the final merger in which the Self ceases to exist, and there is no return to Self (this is called *Nirvikalpa Samadhi*). With our meditative mind, we go beyond time and space, and the possibilities of creating what the mind conceives are infinite.

The purpose of a meditative mind is to know the Unknown, to hear the Unheard and see the Unseen. Tomorrow is my Unseen. Today, I can guess my tomorrow. But if I have a meditative mind, I will know my tomorrow.[7]

[6] Sometimes called *"sushupti"* in Vedic terminology
[7] Yogi Bhajan, April 2, 1979

SADHANA IN THE EARLY MORNING

The Essenes used to roll naked in the morning dew, a practice capable of recharge and rejuvenate the body. It is said that morning dew contained parts of the Cosmic Father and Mother Earth, the union of the two seemingly opposed principles, from which a liquid gold could flow, as it grasps the elusive moment of the first ray of light.[8]

The Native American Pueblo Indians, natives of New Mexico, founded their religion on the contemplation of the rising sun. Mountain Lake says: "We are a population living on top of the world, we are the children of Father Sun, and through our religion, we help Him to go through the sky every day. We do this not just for ourselves but for all the world. If we ceased to practice our religion, in ten years' time, the sun wouldn't rise anymore"[9]

Chinese practitioners of *Qi Gong* (the art of nurturing the vital energy) to practice in the early morning hours. The period from midnight to noon is *Sheng Qi*, meaning "time of the living breath." The best time to practice is around 6:00 in the morning. Early in the morning is like the spring of the day. The winter season of the day, from noon till midnight, is called *Si Qi*, "the time of the dead breath."

---

[8] Meurois-Givaudian, Anne and Daniel *The Other Face of Jesus*
[9] Khalsa, Gobinde Singh, *Diagonal*, year 1, issue 2, June 1986

The seeds planted in spring will bring healthy fruits, while the ones planted in winter are weak and vulnerable. The living breath has its peak at sunrise.[10]

Those who practice Hatha Yoga in different *ashrams* in India generally meditate between 4:00 and 5:00 in the morning and do the physical *asana* work during the next hour. There is a time for everything, and the best time for *sadhana* is the hours before sunrise. It is when the opposites of night and day find balance and the psychic waves are clearest.

With the Adi Mantra, "Ong Namo Guru Dev Namo," we can connect to the Golden Chain of teachers and masters, past and present, and seek their protection. During the *amrit vela*, the magnetic influences of these guides are strongest. During this time, the sun's rays hit the earth at a sixty-degree angle, distributing a higher amount of *praana*, and the body absorbs the energy more efficiently. The lung meridians are more open between 3:00 am to 5:00 am, so breathing control and chanting is easier. The boundaries between the conscious and subconscious minds almost disappear, making it easier to clean and integrate them.

If we meditate at the same time each day, with time, the subconscious supports us and our morning *sadhana* requires less conscious effort. This rhythm becomes natural. By meditating in the *amrit vela*, we process our negativity to cleanse the subconscious. So, instead of encountering fear when we least expect it, allowing it to influence us and cause a reaction, we face our fears in the most neutral way and process it with increasing clarity.

'Amrit Vela Sach Nao Vadiaaee Vichar, Karmee Avay Kapra,
Nadri Mokh Dwar' In the Ambrosial hours before dawn, meditate
on the True Nam and contemplate the Divine Greatness. By the
karma of past actions, the robe of this physical body is obtained,
and, by Divine Grace, the Gate of Liberation is found.'[11]

---

[10] Cohen, Kermeth S. *The Art and Science of Qigong*
[11] Guru Nanak Dev Ji *Japji Sahib*, 4th Pauree

A Good Awakening Starts the Night Before

It is easy to understand that being a *saadhak* depends on your commitment to discipline. However, the commitment extends far beyond the duration of your practice. Getting up before sunrise is a significant change for most people, and it relies on dropping old habits and consciously accepting new ones. When we change when we wake up to a time that we usually are in a deep sleep, we need to adopt new habits. These new habits will not only allow us to awaken easier, but the entire cleaning process triggered by the practice will be more successful.

It is best to go to sleep at least two hours, and preferably four, after our last meal to allow our food to digest. The meal needs to be light, which may mean shifting your main meal to lunchtime. It is advisable to eat your dinner before the sunset.

Prepare to go to sleep by brushing your hair 108 times forward and 108 times backward, with a wooden comb (*kangha*), which does not interfere with your hair's static energy. Hair is like antennae, capable of amplifying your innate intuitive ability and healing power. They extend the magnetic field and are a great source of protein. They synthesize vitamin K through the sunlight, which is vital for us. As yogis, we allow the hair on the body to grow to its natural length. By combing our hair and beard, we eliminate the dust and tangles, which block the energetic flow and our receptive abilities. To finish, wet your fingers with cold water and let them comb through your hair from your temples to the nape of the neck. This will dissipate tension and bring calmness, as well as release residual anger from the day.

Brush your teeth and clean your mouth before bed. We suggest you scrub from the base of your tongue until you feel like gagging so that you can trigger the sputum and the descent of mucus from your nasal passages. Your eyes are going to water, cleaning your tear canals. This procedure cleans the bacteria on your tongue, reducing infections and illnesses.

To relax your body for sleep, refrain from watching screens before going to bed and have a mattress that properly supports your body. There are several yogic practices to prepare us for sleep. Run cold water over your feet for three minutes and then, with a towel, vigorously massage them. Try breathing through your left nostril to calm the body and mind. Be sure to maintain proper hydration by drinking a glass of water before bed. Having committed your day to improve yourself, with gratitude, pray for help to awaken in the morning. Now lie on your right side and sleep.

Yogic technology reveals that if we dwell in spirit, the sun's setting tells us it is time to rest, while if we relate to the animal nature, the setting of the sun is a sign to awaken. The old adage, *early to bed, early to rise, makes a man healthy, wealthy, and wise*, states this same concept – we must prepare to awaken before the sun rises to take advantage of the lifted veil between God and human being.

Morning Routine

How much sleep do you need? The rule of thumb in yoga is, "Eat little, sleep little". However, it is true that the amount of sleep required is different for each person based on their body's needs at different circumstances and stages of life. In general, those regularly doing *sadhana* and practicing Kundalini Yoga require less sleep to feel rested, only 4 ½ to 6 hours. The important aspect is not the time asleep but rather the time in the deep sleep phase. This phase of sleep has few dreams so that body completely recovers in less time. Determine the amount of time to complete your morning routine and set the alarm. To have a calm awakening, consider an alarm that awakens you with music – a mantra or a gentle song. After a while, you may not need an alarm as you automatically wake up at the right time.

Take your time, and try the following sequence before getting out of bed[12]:

---

[12] Physical Wisdom, published by KRI 1997

Wake Up Series

- Lie on your back and stretch your arms over your head; at the same time, straighten your legs down, letting your back and rib cage find their natural alignment. This helps restore your magnetic field and awaken the body.

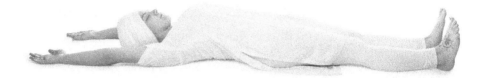

- Before opening the eyes, cup the hands over the eyes. As you draw your hands away from the face allow light filter gradually through your fingers. Massage your face, hair, and beard.

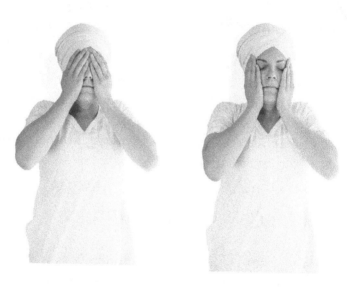

- This is the perfect moment for Stretch Pose. Let the soft support of the bed help to hold the position. It feels wonderful! Practice this position with a minute of Breath of Fire.

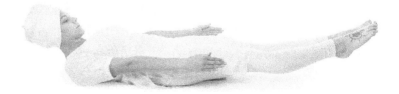

- Rub the palms of your hands and the soles of your feet together vigorously.

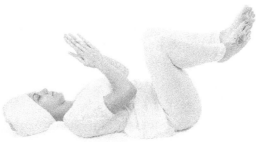

- Hug the knees to your chest and roll up. Come into Baby (Child) Pose. Imagine you have a long and heavy tail and move from left to right. Shake it strongly. Coordinate the breath with the movement, inhale to the left, exhale to the right. This movement aligns the lumbar and sacral parts of your spine and eliminates gases, stimulating the *apana*, the elimination process.

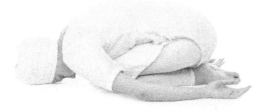

- You are now ready to get out of bed and make your way to the bathroom.

It is beneficial for men to urinate *seated*, blocking and releasing the urine flow four to five times. Emptying your bladder completely in this way prevents gallstones and prostate problems later in life. Urinating applying Kegel exercises helps women as well, reinforcing the pelvic floor and helping to prevent incontinence and other health issues later in life.

Ishnaan Hydrotherapy

It is time for *ishnaan* hydrotherapy, in other words, a cold shower! Ishnaan is the use of cold water to help the body heal itself. "Ish" literally means illness; "naan" means "does not exist." Water as a therapy has been widely used in the past as a scientific, religious, and yogic modality. In the eighteenth and nineteenth centuries, doctors would suggest cold baths in the North Sea to patients with psychiatric problems. It is widely believed that bathing in rivers considered holy, like the Nile in Egypt or the Ganges in India, is a cure for many illnesses. Even today, people bathe in the sacred tank of Amritsar at the Golden Temple to heal and purity themselves.

Bathing in cold water in the morning is an important part of a successful *sadhana*. Cold water on the skin invigorates the circulation, creating blood flow and waking up the entire physiology. One modern medical use of cold water is treating the risk of hematoma from inflammation and bruises caused by trauma. The application of cold water shrinks the blood vessels and prevents the stagnation of blood.

It is important to note that warm water is the treatment for some medical conditions. Some examples are the treatment for cold or flu, major circulatory problems like Reynaud's Syndrome, severe cardiac problems, or during pregnancy or menstruation. Those suffering from high blood pressure and sciatica also need to be cautious, gradually changing from warm water to cold water. If you are uncertain, always check with your medical advisor.

Apart from these situations, the cold water forces the blood to reach all the extremities to warm up the body. The blood, going externally, applies some pressure on the internal organs provoking a blood reflow. By increasing the amount of blood in the skin, the whole system becomes more sensitive and alert. The stimulation of the glands, guardians of our health, produces a better resistance to illness while the increased circulation flushes our liver and kidneys. Our body is stronger, and we are in an optimum state for meditation.

There is a complete process in yogic technology to prepare for the cold water, rather than jumping directly into a cold shower. The first step is to massage the body using a little almond or sesame oil. This practice benefits the nervous system. To protect the sensitive areas around the sexual organs and inner thigh, both men and women wear shorts or *kachera*, the thigh-length underwear of the Sikhs, in the shower. Step into the shower, let the water hit the extremities – arms and legs first, then onto the body. Vigorously massage the body to stimulate circulation and stay under the cold water as long as you can. Some people find it beneficial to briefly remain under the cold water, get out and massage the body, and reenter the water. After four or five times, the cold water will feel pleasant. When finished, the last step is to dry the body, rubbing vigorously with a towel to aid in circulation. For those having great difficulty with cold water, start slowly and build up over time.

We comb our hair in the same way as before going to sleep and then tie it on the top of our head where the *Shashara*, the seventh chakra, is located. Placing the hair there pulls the energy upward, believed to support the connection with our Infinite Self. We cover the hair with a turban[13] or any headcover made of cotton, preferably white, to keep the energy stable during yoga and meditation.

After drinking three or four glasses of either warm water or lemon water, we are ready for *sadhana*! But before really starting our spiritual practice each day, we can look in the mirror and remind ourselves that we are not the doer. The Universe has us covered.

---

[13] Note that certain turban styles hold the twenty-six cranial bones in right position. As with all yogic lifestyle suggestions, try this and experience if there is a difference.

CHALLENGES TO A SUCCESSFUL SADHANA

Resistances are challenges in our lives that come when we oppose the natural flow of things – when we oppose the *hukam*, Divine Will. Resistance creates a conflict that causes an emotional imbalance. Negative judgment of the past sometimes gives rise to resistance, influencing the present experience. Holding the memory, we feel sad or upset. One way to get through resistance is to surrender to it and, in that way, remove its power. If we surrender to a feeling of sadness rather than fearing it, we may result in some pleasant feelings, even gratitude. If we resist, we fear the future, whereas the future unfolds with ease if we surrender. Surrendering is the opposite of resisting, and it is the path to happiness. Yogi Bhajan once wrote to me and said, "Not accepting what God has given us is to be anti-God. Rejecting Him is to challenge our own soul."

It is difficult to sit and meditate at the same time each day, every day, and so the discipline of *sadhana* creates resistance. We want to meditate only when we feel like it, not daily. The truth is that we give too much importance to our moods. They are superficial and variable and can be nothing more than a resistance. If we practice only when we are in the mood, we make our connection to our Infinite Self, God, dependent on external conditions. We are valuing the "me status" higher than the Infinite One. At this point, our discipline serves us. It supports us even at the worst time. When our feelings and emotions put up a resistance, it is simple, relax and surrender to discipline. *Keep up, and you will be kept up.* Do not evaluate the practice, meditation, and prayers from the feelings and emotions you have in that precise moment. Keep going and assess the effects that gradually come to your life, character, and relationships. In the spiritual life, what is important is perseverance through change, time, and processes.

Sources of Strength for a Consistent Sadhana

When we feel down, lack strength, our minds wander and we find it hard to focus, it's good to remember there is a large energy reservoir within us. It is the *Manipura,* the third chakra at the navel. All yoga starts from the navel center. *Manipura* represents the strength of the spiritual warrior, who knows their mission and acts fearlessly from their essence. The lotus representing it has ten petals, the number ten represents completeness – the number one represents the sense of self and zero represents the Infinite Self. A person with mastery over the third chakra knows how to start and complete an action. Together with the first and second chakras, the third chakra forms an energy triangle that guides the action, completing the conceptualization. Work on the third chakra helps our determination and reconciles our practice.

Every practitioner on the spiritual path at some point encounters a time of crisis that is more than a lack of energy or motivation. There is a stalemate with the ego as the antagonist, motivated by its desire for happiness. Because we have an ego, the search for happiness is a dilemma for every human being. Society reinforces the quest for the elusive state of happiness. The fear of not realizing happiness pushes us to satisfy our desires for momentary satisfactions, drops of water for our thirsty ego. It is not easy to accept that discipline and commitment are the way to genuine fulfillment. The ego starts resisting. This is Shakti Pad, one of the five phases on the path to wisdom[14].

There is no way around the pit of Shakti Pad. The *saadhak* must climb through the depth of one's own doubt in order to commit to the spiritual path of happiness, *Dharma.* Like a teenager, we may want to make choices without the burden of responsibility or the implication of commitment. It is a mistake to choose a more stimulating path than to remain steadfast to the goal that we have already started towards – self-identity.

Commitment is the key to release doubt, but the attachment to ego is strong. It is the eternal dilemma "to be or not to be" instead of the simple "to be, to be[15]." Surrendering to the discipline of commitment focused on the goal requires an

---

14 Aquarian Teacher Level One Textbook
15 Aquarian Teacher Level One Textbook, p.8

absence of doubt that awakens a realization of God's will and an acceptance of our divine identity.

The Power of Prayer

No longer bound by ego, we experience divinity. How can we choose between desires, needs, and that so hard to grasp Divine will? We could practice all the yoga in the world and still not free ourselves from the grasp of ego. This is when we need our greatest power, the power of prayer.

The arc line is the part of our electromagnetic field that extends from ear to ear, across the hairline and the brow, like a halo. It is the center of the aura and our connection to the Divine. An effective way of clearing the arc line is to connect intentionally with the Infinite; we call this mental effort prayer. We are accustomed to understand prayer it as a request for something, addressed to the Infinite. Regarding prayer, the Archbishop Anthony Bloom says, "Sit down and don't do anything, just sit in front of God." This silent sitting before the Infinite or anyway you believe is contact with God, is prayer. The action of projecting yourself externally to the Infinite, doing it from the arc line, which has a vast energetic impact. Mentally, prayer involves the passage through the neutral mind and making a connection with the Universal Mind. The more intense and stable the connection, the more transcendent the personal consciousness of the prayer and therefore the more effective it is.

Conflicting thoughts dim our projection and we may feel that our prayers do not work. The neutral mind is capable of projecting the soul's impulses to the universe in prayer. Prayer is a journey of discovery, we can learn. As Christian, Sikh, or any other religion, our prayer is a dialogue with God, contact with the Infinite, the Universal Consciousness. Prayer requires discipline. Father Andrew said, "Prayer is you praying, it is not something external to you."

Kundalini Yoga technology teaches us that prayer is not trying to establish a connection with our soul, but remembering that connection, which is always there. It is not talking to a God that exists outside of our own innate Divinity. Prayer is to enter into contact with the Unknown Self while unifying it with our known self. This union makes God alive in us, awakened, not longer sleeping. Our greatest tool and our greatest power is prayer. It takes us beyond human suffering. We become humble and innocent and the presence of the Unknown in us washes away everything. With this power, we can fulfill or destiny.

Therefore, we pray at the end of *sadhana*.

Mantra, Naad, and the Yoga of the Mind

The whole of creation originated from the sound. Human creatures come from that original vibration and remain connected through the spirit that animated them. Humans' search for freedom derives from a longing caused by the separation from that vibration. This creates a need to reunite with the original vibration, with the Naam — to synchronize with this constant vibration that supports the universe.

"In the beginning, there was the Word. And the Word was with God.
And the Word was God."

The Holy Bible (John, 1:1).

If we understand the Word as a projection of thought, we enter the theory of *mantra* as an expression of the projection in sound and vibration. The etymological meaning of mantra is *MAN* – "mind" and *TRA* – "projection wave." Therefore, mantra is a projection of the mind, a wave frequency that retrains the psyche. A more yogic understanding of the word is *MAN* – "mind" or "now," *TA* – "life," and *RA-* "sun," meaning "synchronizing the mind in the present moment with a radiant life."

A *mantra* is a group of letters or words with a specific meaning or mental projection that creates sound. More important than the meaning of the words is the experience that it generates. Ancient yogis, while in a state of high consciousness, expressed sounds. Now when we chant these sounds, we can experience the same level of consciousness. *Mantra* awakens the memory of who and what we are. It works like a pair of scissors and vertically cuts the flow of images and thoughts moving through the mind. Through *mantra*, the negative and positive minds come to a resolution through the neutral and Universal mind and transform obstructive mental states.

When we chant a *mantra*, the vibrational effect results from the tongue's movement touching meridian points on the palate affecting the hypothalamus, which controls the autonomic nervous system. The more we focus on the vibration of the *mantra*, the greater the effect. It is self-reflexology.

The best practice is to consciously vibrate the sound of the mantra and simultaneously listen to the sound. Sound is a wave that we can hear; the tiniest sound humans hear is sixty vibrations per second. However, when we listen deeply with sympathetic resonance, we can hear all sounds, even the sound of atoms and light. Sound is a connection between the individual consciousness and the Universal consciousness, a link between the manifested and unmanifested.

Sound created all existence, the entire universe. Scientific experiments have shown that some sounds create specific forms and images[16], which remind us of the organic structure of human beings and plants. In one experiment, chanting the sound OM reproduced the image of OM in its original language.

Most *mantras* used in Kundalini Yogi are in Gurmukhi – the language of the Sikh Gurus, while others are in Sanskrit and sometimes in Western languages[17]. In our practice, when we repeat a mantra aloud consciously that is called *jaap*, and when we mentally recite a mantra, it is called *Simran*. Either way, with prayerful intention and discipline, the restorative healing power of mantra is effective.

Japji Sahib

Aquarian Sadhana begins with the recitation of *Japji Sahib* (meditation on the soul), the beautiful prayer written in the mid-fifteenth century by Guru Nanak Dev Ji, the first Sikh Guru. Five hundred years ago, Guru Nanak said there is One

---

16 https://en.wikipedia.org/wiki/Cymatics
17 A unique feature of Kundalini Yoga as taught by Yogi Bhajan® is the use of mantras from the Sikh tradition and also the use of western words and affirmations.

God, one Supreme Truth, called different names by believers of different faiths. Guru Nanak's teachings revealed a state of absolute neutrality. He is a perfect example of an enlightened spiritual man and, at the same time, a householder with a family and a job. This was revolutionary at the time because the ascetics were convinced of the need to renounce all attachments to everyday life in order to be spiritually elevated.

In the forty *paurees* or verses of *Japji Sahib*, he describes the steps to liberation from the cycle of birth and death for people of all faiths, then and even now. Thus, I advise all students and teachers of Kundalini Yoga to read *Japji Sahib* to experience this holy prayer's enormous transformational power.

Japji Sahib's effectiveness is understood through the science of Naad Yoga, the yoga of sound, capable of bringing energetic and physical changes to the individual who consciously vibrates it. In *Japji Sahib*, Guru Nanak proclaims the union of the soul with the Beloved, the relationship between a human being and the Infinite. It is traditional to honor the wisdom of *Japji Sahib* by covering our head when we read or recite it, and when not in use, keeping its written form covered with a clean cloth and not placing it directly on the ground.

Japji Sahib begins with the *Mul Mantra*. It is said that the entire wisdom of the *Japji Sahib* can be found in understanding the *Mul Mantra*, so this mantra is meditated upon on its own – *Ek Ong Kaar, Sat Naam, Kartaa Purkh, Nirbao, Nirvair, Akal Murat, Ajoonee Saibang, Gurprasaad, Jaap, Aad Sach, Jugaad Sach Hai Bhee Sach, Naanak Ho See Bhee Sach.*

Japji is a complete system of healing and transformation. Like our human form, it is built from the five elements of the universe – earth, water, fire, air, and ether. When we recite it, the five elements stimulate our chakras. Starting with the *Mul Mantra*, it aligns with the aura and the eight chakras and moves sequentially down through our body's centers of energy. It is a journey to shed negative habits and to develop proportional intelligence and consciousness.

When recited, each of the forty paurees (*Mul Mantra*, thirty-eight verses, and the *Shalok*) generates a specific effect. Yogi Bhajan gave the transformational effects of chanting each *pauree* of *Japji Sahib* as a meditation of its own. Chant a specific *pauree* eleven times a day and experience the power of the *Shabd Guru*.[18]

---

[18] Taken from "Psyche of the Soul – The Nit Naym Banis, with additional Shabds and prayers, and their effects," by Siri Singh Sahib Bhai Sahib Harbhajan Singh Khalsa Yogiji and Bhai Sahiba Sardarni Sahiba Bibiji Inderjit Kaur Khalsa

THE EXPERIENCE OF AQUARIAN SADHANA

Aquarian Sadhana is one tenth of our day, two and a half hours. The first part of this form of *sadhana* is the recitation of Japji Sahib, which takes around 20 minutes. In addition to the remarkable effects produced by every single pauree or stanza, these forty steps lead us immediately to a different state of consciousness, changing our vibration and opening us to the benefits of the yoga and meditation that follow.

We begin the yoga practice with flexibility postures to prepare the physical body and then practice a kriya for about an hour, including relaxation. If the relaxation is not included in the kriya, add a seven to fifteen minutes relaxation at the end of the kriya. Any yoga set that fits in the time period works for *sadhana*. I recommend kriyas, which work on the spine, or the nervous or glandular systems. Choose kriyas that you know how to practice, as well as having guidance from a certified teacher.

Next is sixty-two minutes of specific meditations (that will be described later), followed by the long Time Sun Song and a prayer. This is the classic structure of *Aquarian Sadhana* as we practice in Kundalini Yoga. Remember that any regular spiritual practice is *sadhana*, and therefore we can structure a *sadhana* of our own. In our tradition, the *Aquarian Sadhana* supports us during the transition into the Age of Aquarius.

While any *sadhana* is highly beneficial, *sadhana* practiced in a group multiplies the practice's strength exponentially. It can synchronize each individual to a shared vibratory frequency, despite each person initially being in a different energetic state. The individual consciousness fuses with group consciousness, and the individual aura itself merges into a unique collective aura. Working together toward the same objective helps transcend ego identification in favor of sharing, interchange, and communication. Group practice is so important and powerful that we suggest that if you are unable to physically practice with a group or online that you imagine being with other people, hear them chanting and chant with them.

If two and half hours is too daunting a commitment, begin by practicing however long is possible. With patience, you find yourself going to bed earlier, sleeping profoundly, and awakening earlier so that you can extend the duration of practice. Do your best, with sincerity and devotion, and witness the results. The self-discipline of *sadhana* carries through the rest of the day and is a powerful component of self-realization.

Physical Preparation and the Importance of Working on Your Body

Kundalini Yoga is a complete yoga and is extremely efficient. It has a solid scientific base. Often challenging, it asks for commitment but grants us a proportional result. With its methodology to strengthen and balance our physical systems, yoga lets the energy flow within our bodies through the non-anatomic pathways called *meridians* or *nadis*. Yogic *mudras* and postures stimulate the energy *meridians* in the body. As mudras and postures are perfected and the energy unblocked, *praana* flows with ease.

For the best effect, we take the time to prepare the body before we sit for *sadhana*. During the practice, it is important to be aware of our body, resulting in a more pleasant experience. Little by little, work to increase your joints and muscles' flexibility and decrease the discomfort when in Easy Pose or holding a posture for a length of time. Recognize when a position is not suitable for your body at this time. "Stretching" means to expand the possibilities of movement, elasticity, and flexibility of the body. Never use force to stretch further, instead relax into it and release it so that your muscles remember their real nature, which is forgotten due to tension and bad habits. When the strings of a musical instrument are too loose, they do not produce the intended sounds; when they are too tense, they may break. This helps us to understand the needs of our muscles and joints.

As children, our bones are softer, and they are extremely loose, preventing injuries. As we age, our bodies get tense, and our muscles lock up, so when we fall, we are injured. When our body is flexible, the risk of injury is significantly reduced. Both stretching and relaxation are essential to the body; it is a law of balance. As yogis, upon awakening, we do not immediately jump out of bed; instead, first, we awaken the body with breathing and stretching as described in the Wake-Up Series. Our body needs kindness; it is difficult for our body to go from a sleeping state directly to an activity state, and, surely you have noticed, neither can the mind.

Waking the body up gradually is an act of love toward our body and a step toward consciousness. Our body has a connection to our soul and our mind. As our boundary, it is an image of ourselves and a tool to experience the world on the physical level.

Environment

The physical environment is essential to encourage relaxation and an openness to work on ourselves. It is good to meditate not only at the same time but also in the same place. Because clothes absorb energy, it is best to wear clothes not worn during the day or for sleep but reserved for *sadhana*. This also applies to the mat, blankets, or shawls used in *sadhana*. It is best to use a mat made of wool or animal skin to insulate the body from the ground and separate our magnetic field from that of the Earth.

Keep a serene environment. Consider all of the senses when setting up the space. First, be sure that it is clean and pleasing to the eye. Let the air circulate so that it is always fresh and pleasant to breathe. Keep the temperature neither too hot nor too cold so that our muscles, circulation, and concentration can work at their best. Energetically, the space will become like a temple, a graceful place where we can connect with ourselves.

Some authors place additional restrictions on the place you practice *sadhana*, such as locking the door to prevent anyone from coming into the space. I encourage you to open your door to your spouse and your children so that they enjoy the benefits of *sadhana* and improve your relationships. Invite anybody who is interested, as we all benefit from group *sadhana*.

If you have the opportunity to practice in nature, on top of a mountain, by the sea, near a waterfall, or on the banks of a river, do it because the energetic vibrations of these natural places strengthen the practice. Similarly, if you find yourself in a new place where the energy feels negative or stagnate, you can purify the energy. One method to change the vibration in a room is to walk clockwise around the room's perimeter eleven times, chanting the mantra "*Har - Haray - Haree - Whaa-Hay - Guroo*". Vibrate one sound on each step, completing the mantra every six steps. If there are other people with you, they sit in the center of the room, chanting the mantra with their hands in front of the navel, palms facing the body with the left hand closer than the right hand. Without touching each other or the body, one hand moves upward while the other moves downward; the whole movement is about 10 inches. (Guru Dev Singh, Assisi 1999).

Relaxation

Relaxation is a widely used term, and yet few people really experience it. Relaxing is a natural gift. A state of inaction benefits the whole body. Our intention is not simply to release physical tensions but also to calm the mind to have both a relaxed body and an attentive mind. With societal pressure to be active and achieve success, voluntary passiveness appears counterproductive. However, we discover that the more we relax, the more we realize body awareness and tap its full vitality; the state of passive relaxation is essential.

Every tension in the body represents an energetic block impeding the flow of praana in both the psychic and physical functions. How do we, as yogis, utilize relaxation? There are short rests in in every Kundalini Yoga class after an exercise or a group of exercises, unless otherwise instructed. Each class includes a deep relaxation. This relaxation is always after the physical kriya because after releasing muscular tension, it is easier for the body to relax. This deep relaxation is as important as the kriya and meditation, and actually necessary for the body to assimilate their effects. The organs, cells and tissues and the brain are able to regenerate as needed. Relaxation is an essential aid to restore our energy in a brief amount of time.

Aquarian Sadhana Meditation

Yogi Bhajan gave the following meditation for the Aquarian *Sadhana* on June 21, 1992, to support us in the transition into the Aquarian Age. This sixty-two-minute meditative practice consists of seven meditations in a precise order, each with a specific length of time.

1. *The Adi Shakti Mantra* (7 minutes)

Ek Ong Kaar Sat Naam Siree Whaa-hay Guroo

*"The One Creator created this creation. Truth is His Name.
Great beyond description is His Infinite Wisdom"*

Known as "Long Ek Ong Kaars" or "Morning Call", this mantra comes from Baba Siri Chand (1494-1629), the son of Guru Nanak. It is the foundation of the Aquarian *Sadhana* meditation and is chanted without musical accompaniment (the other six mantras may be sung with or without musical accompaniment).

This meditation has eight parts (*ashtang mantra*) with a precise breath and rhythm done in two and a half breaths. On the first deep inhalation, chant a short *Ek*, then *Ong* and *Kaar* are equal length to complete the exhalation. On the second deep inhalation, chant a short *Sat*, then a long *Naam*, and on the last bit of breath, chant *Siri*. *Naam* is the same length as *Ong* and *Kaar* together. Now, take a half inhalation and chant *Whaa-hay Guru*. This phrase is the length of *Ong*.

For each sound, visualize as follows[19]:

- *Ek* - Focus on and contract the first chakra, the anus. Visualize the entire Universe within your being.

- *Ong* - Focus on and contract the second chakra, the sexual organs. Visualize the creative power of all the creation.

- *Kaar* - Focus on and contract the third chakra, the navel, and draw it back towards the spine. Visualize the sun, the moon, and the stars reflecting light on you.

- *Sat* - Focus on the fourth chakra, the heart. Raise the diaphragm and the solar plexus and visualize your illumination.

[19] A Year with the Master, pp63

102

- *Naam* - Focus on the fifth chakra, the throat, and apply a slight neck lock (*Jalandara Bhanda*). Feel that you fully exist within your humility.

- *Siree* - Focus on the sixth chakra, the third eye. Acknowledge the miracle of the creation and the Creator.

- *Whaa-hay* - Focus on the seventh chakra, the crown and draw the energy to the top of the head. Visualize the energy falling around you in ecstasy while chanting *Hay*.

- *Guroo* - Focus on the eighth chakra, the aura, and totally defuse your energy into the Infinite.

Relax as the mantra completes the cycle and inhale deeply to start again.

This meditation opens and balances the chakras and can change the arc line and one's destiny. This is the first mantra taught by Yogi Bhajan during his first year in America. During those early years, it was chanted in morning *sadhana* for 62 minutes and sometimes for two and a half hours. It is said to open the lock at the solar plexus to open one's heart center and connect you directly to the all-creating and stimulating energy: the Kundalini.

2. *Waah Yantee, Kaar Yantee* (7 minutes)

Waah Yantee, Kaar Yantee	Great Macro-self. Creative Self
Jagadootpatee	All that is creative through time.
Aadak It Whaa-haa	All that is the Great One.
Brahmaaday Trayshaa Guroo	Three aspects of God – Brahma, Vishnu, Mahesh
It Whaa-hay Guroo	That is Whaa hay Guroo.

Using the ancient words of Patanjali, this mantra stimulates the heart chakra and balances the ethereal bodies. In the space beyond time and duality, this mantra vibrates with all the power of centuries of prayers. It connects you to the source of everything by stimulating the radiance of the Self. It leads you beyond time and space, as the consciousness expands beyond the trinity-guru of Brahma (the creator), Vishnu (the sustainer), and Shiva (the destroyer).

3. *Mul Mantra* (7 minutes)

Ek Ong Kaar	One Creator. Creation
Sat Naam	Truth Identified (Named)
Kartaa Purkh	Doer of Everything
Nirbho	Fearless
Nirvair	Without Revenge
Akaal Moorat	Undying
Ajoonee	Unborn
Saibung	Self-illumined. Self-existent
Gurprasaad	By the Guru's Grace
Jap	Chant!
Aad Such	True in the beginning
Jugaad Such	True through all time
Hai Bhee Such	True eve now
Nanak Hosee Bhee Such	Nanak says, Truth shall ever be.

As discussed before *Mul Mantra (root mantra)* is the opening passage of *Japji Sahib*, as well as the *mangla charan*, beginning prayer, of the *Siri Guru Granth Sahib* ji. In *Mul Mantra*, Guru Nanak reveals the essential belief of Sikhs, a declaration of God as One. Here, Nanak describes the Divine One who is beyond time and space. This Divinity is the principle of Truth. A person, who understands his own nature, acknowledging it in unity with the Absolute, aligns his will with the will of God. Aligned with *Hukam*, the will of God, through *dharma*, all karma brought into this life is dissolved. The *Mul Mantra* opens the flow of the Universal Consciousness.

This mantra consists of 108 letters. Traditionally 108 is a sacred number, the number of completion. The *Mul Mantra* heals depression and feelings of inadequacy and insecurity. The power of this mantra lies in the *Naam* because we find the essence and the basis of all other mantras in it.

The *Mul Mantra* tells us One Creator created us, and we are one with Him. When we experience this reality, we know that our identity is *Sat Naam. Naam* is not a word; it is a vibration not created by humans. It is unique. It is creativity itself. The Creator is not separate from His creation; He is within it. Once we experience this reality and are one with everything, how can we fear that someone might hurt us or take something from us? This realization leads us to reject asceticism because we believe God is everywhere and in all things, so we do not need to flee from others or society. In this Divine Energy, everything is still, already existing, and eternal. Embodying this reality, all suffering departs. By finding this energy within us, we can understand how He is eternal, never subject to change. Everything rotates around this Divine Energy. Its essence is the Truth – it was in the beginning, it is now, and it will always be.

4. *Sat Siri, Siri Akal* (7 minutes)

Sat Siree	Great Truth
Siree Akaal	Respected Immortal
Siree Akaal	Respected Immortal
Mahaa Akaal	Great Deathless
Mahaa Akaal	Great Deathless
Sat Naam	Truth Identified (Named)
Akaal Moorat	Deathless Image of God
Whaa-hay Guroo	Great beyond description is His Wisdom

This *ashtang mantra*, given by Guru Gobind Singh (1666-1708), a spiritual warrior and the tenth Guru of the Sikhs, is considered the mantra of the Aquarian Age. Beyond the literal meaning, its frequency helps us transition from the Piscean Age to the Aquarian Age.

We are truly free when we know *akaal*, the undying, the ecstatic state where the ego has no reason to exist. To become a tree, the seed has to die. It has to become nothing and therefore becomes part of the tree[20]. This state allows us to be new every day. When we are nothing, God is there. This is *shuniya*, the empty space of when we die while yet alive.

---

[20] "Truly, truly, I say to you, unless a grain of wheat falls into the earth and dies, it remains alone; but if it dies, it bears much fruit." The Holy Bible, John 12:24

5. *Rakhay Rakhan Haar* (7 minutes)

Rakhay Rakhanhaar Aap Ubaariun

You who saves, save us all and take us across.

Gur Kee Pairee Paa-eh Kaaj Savaariun

Uplifting and giving the excellence,

*Hoaa Aap Dayaal Manho
Na Visaariun*

You gave us the touch of the lotus feet of the Guru and all our jobs are done.

*Saadh Janaa Kai Sung
Bhavjal Taariun*

You have become merciful, kind, and compassionate, and so our mind does not forget You.

*Saakat Nindak Dusht Khin
Maa-eh Bidaariun*

In the company of the holy beings, you save us from misfortune and calamities, scandals, and disrepute.

*Tis Sahib Kee Tayk Naanak
Mania Maa-eh*

Godless and slanderous enemies – You finish them in timelessness.
That great Lord is my anchor.

*Jis Simrat Sukh Ho-eh Saglay Dookh
Jaa-eh.*

Nanak, keep firm in your mind by meditating and repeating His Name. All happiness comes and all sorrows and pain go away.

Rakhay Rakhanhaar is a beautiful *shabd* composed by Guru Arjan Dev (1563 - 1606), the son of Guru Ram Das and the fifth Sikh Guru. It is part of the *Rehras Sahib*, the evening prayer of the Sikhs, which includes the writings of Guru Nanak Dev, Guru Amar Das, Guru Ram Das, Guru Arjan Dev, and Guru Gobind Singh. Guru Arjan Dev collected the hymns of his predecessors and other saints and sages of different religions, together with his compositions to form the *Siri Guru Granth Sahib*, the living Guru of the Sikh for now and all time.

With our faith in the unknown strengthened and immortality realized, this *shabd* shelters and protects us, defeating the enemies – doubt and fear. In this process, we find humility and faith, letting us manifest the Divine Self and become true disciples of the eternal Guru within.

6. *Whaa-hay Guroo, Whaa-hay Jeeo* (22 minutes)

Waa-hay Guroo, Whaa-hay Guroo, Whaa-hay Guroo, Whaa-hay Jeeo

"Waa-hay Guroo" is an expression of ecstasy for which there is no real translation. You could say, *"Indescribably great is His Infinity, Ultimate, Wisdom."*[21]

This is the mantra of ecstasy. We chant this mantra in *virasana*, Hero or Warrior Pose, like a spiritual warrior, preparing for the battle and assured of victory. We accept our challenges, loving and acknowledging them as opportunities for growth, as well as paths to expansion and prosperity. We evoke the power to serve and honor our soul. To practice, sit on the left heel, place the right foot next to the left leg. The right knee is up near the chest. Ideally, the left heel is on the perineum close to the anus. The spine is straight and in neck lock. The hands are in Prayer Pose at the Heart Center. Eyes are focused at the tip of the nose.

7. *Guroo Guroo Whaa-hay Guroo, Guroo Raam Das Guroo* (5 minutes)

This is the beautiful mantra of Guru Ram Das, the Guru of tolerance, healing, and love. Through our connection to the Golden Chain, he continues to serve and protect all those who walk this spiritual path. With the humility and sweetness of *bhakti* (devotion), the spiritual warrior's conscience obtains balance. Without Bhakti, there is no *Shakti* (spiritual power).

[21] Aquarian Teacher Level One Textbook, pp 153

Kriya the Essence of Self

July, 1985

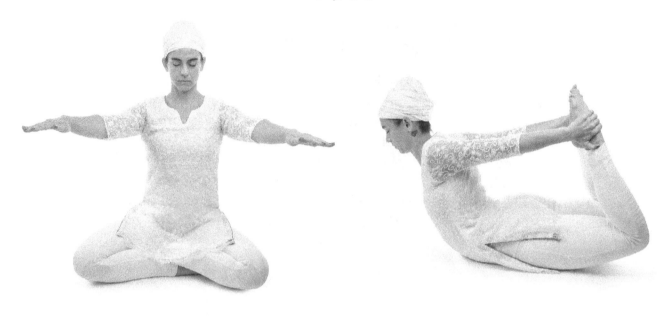

PART ONE

Time: 4 Minutes

Sit in Easy Pose with a straight spine. Extend the arms forward and out to 60 degrees, parallel to the ground, elbows straight, palms face down. Move the arms from the shoulders in backward small circles with Breath of Fire. Gradually increase the power of the breath and move the arms wider and faster for the duration. Continue for 4 minutes.

Comments: For the best results, practice this exercise very energetically. The faster the breath is, the more powerfully it stimulates the heart.

PART TWO

Time: 1 Minute

Lie on the stomach, bend the knees and grasp the ankles, come up into Bow Pose. Rock forward and back from the shoulders to the knees. Coordinate the rocking motion with a powerful Breath of Fire, so powerful it feels as though fire is coming from the nostrils. Continue for 1 minute.

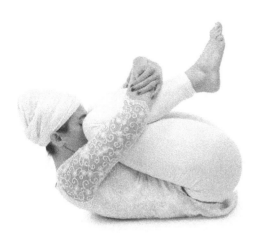

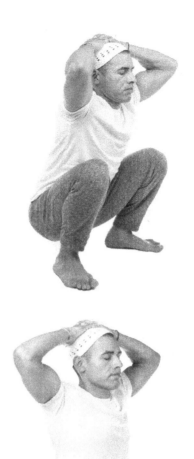

PART THREE

Time: 1 ½ Minutes

Lie on the back, bend the knees into the chest, wrap the arms around the knees, bringing the forehead toward the knees. Rock forward and back on the entire length of the spine. Coordinate the rocking motion with Breath of Fire. Continue for 1 ½ minutes.

PART FOUR

26 Repetitions

Squat with the feet wide apart, knees drawn into the chest and the heels flat on the ground, Crow Pose. Clasp the hands in Venus Lock on top of the head, keep the spine straight with a gentle neck lock. Inhale, rise up to standing, exhale return to Crow Pose. Repeat this movement for a total of 26 repetitions. (In the original class Yogi Bhajan counted to keep the students together at a specific pace – 1 rising up and 2 coming down into Crow Pose.)

PART FIVE

Time: 2 Minutes

Repeat Part One for 2 minutes.

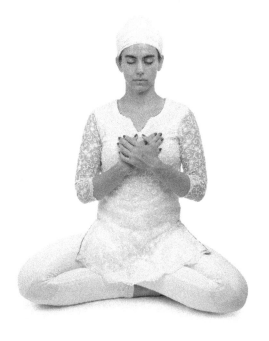

PART SIX

Time: 11-31 Minutes

Sit in Easy Pose with a straight spine. Place one hand over the other at the Heart Center. Close the eyes. Drop any self-limitations; surrender the self to the Self. In this expanded awareness, experience your essence. Remain focused and meditate for 11-31 minutes. Musical variation: Play *Dhan Dhan Ram Das Guru (The Blessing)* by Sangeet Kaur. Sing with the music, beam from the heart. Call out to Guru Ram Das to open the heart and create a miracle in your life.

Comments: When you are weighed down by the scars and disappointments of life it is difficult to sense the broader reality of which you are a part. The pains create blocks to the inflow of cosmic energy and you become less sensitive to your own possibilities. This series guides the *praana* through the body to the heart chakra, "opening" the heart so you can give and receive love without fear, anger, or resentment and experience compassion. In this state of compassion, you release the pain of former relationships, energize current relationships on a higher level and begin to express your divine essence. The exercises in this kriya release tension strengthen the digestion and open the lungs.

First Plane Meditation

February 23, 1976

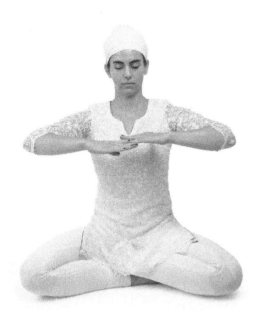

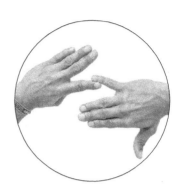

Time: 11 minutes, gradually build to 31 minutes maximum.

Sit in Easy pose with a straight spine. Raise the elbows out to the sides, forearms parallel to the ground, hands in front of the heart center. Palms face down and the left hand is closer to the body than the right. The right thumb is tucked under but not touches the right palm. The inner side of the first digit of the right index finger touches the inner side of the first digit of the left little finger. These two fingers are angled 45 degrees away from the rest of the fingers on their respective hands. The left thumb stretches out towards the body and slightly upward. The right middle, ring and little fingers are held straight and together. The left

index, middle and ring fingers are held straight and together. There is no bend in the wrist. Close the eyes.

Inhale deeply and chant GOBINDAY, GOBINDAY, GOBINDAY, GOBINDAY, GOBINDAY, GOBINDAY, GOBIND-AH, four repetitions of the complete mantra on each breath. Each cycle takes about 11 seconds. With practice you may increase to 5 repetitions per breath.

Comments: This is a powerful but subtle meditation. This meditation requires practice to be able to hold the mudra and also have enough breath to complete four repetitions of the mantra. It affects a meridian in the arm that affects the brain

Kriya for the Instinctual Self

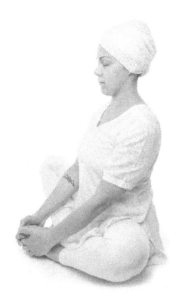 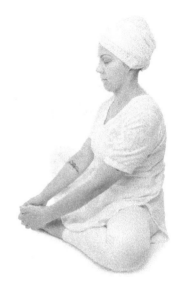

PART ONE

Time: 1-3 Minutes

Sit with the soles of the feet pressed together. Grab the feet with both hands and draw them into the groin, keeping the knees as close to the floor as possible. Inhale and flex the spine forward. Exhale and flex the spine back. Keep the head level and straight. Create a steady rhythm, coordinating the movement with the breath.

Continue for 1-3 minutes.

To End: Inhale, hold the breath briefly, exhale and relax.

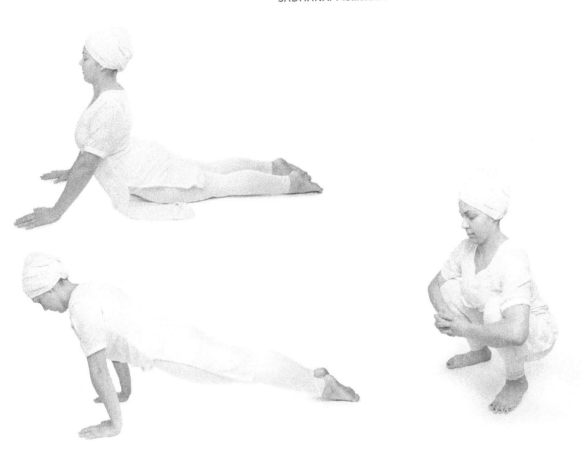

PART TWO

Time: 1-3 Minutes

Lie on the stomach, place hands under the shoulders with palms flat. Elongate the spine, lift the head, chest and heart up, drop the shoulders, stretch the head up and back. Straighten the arms gradually, without straining, into Cobra Pose.

Inhale and raise the buttocks so that the body forms a straight line from the head to the toes, tops of the feet are on the ground, Plank Pose. Exhale and lower the body back into Cobra Pose.

Continue rhythmically with powerful breathing for 1-3 minutes.

To End: Inhale in Cobra Pose, briefly suspend the breath, apply *Mul Bandh*. Exhale and relax.

PART THREE

Time: 1-3 Minutes

Squat with the feet wide apart, knees drawn into the chest and the heels flat on the ground, Crow Pose. Keep the spine straight with a gentle neck lock. Wrap the arms around the knees with the fingers interlocked in Venus Lock. Breathe Breath of Fire.

Continue for 1-3 minutes.

To End: Inhale, exhale and relax.

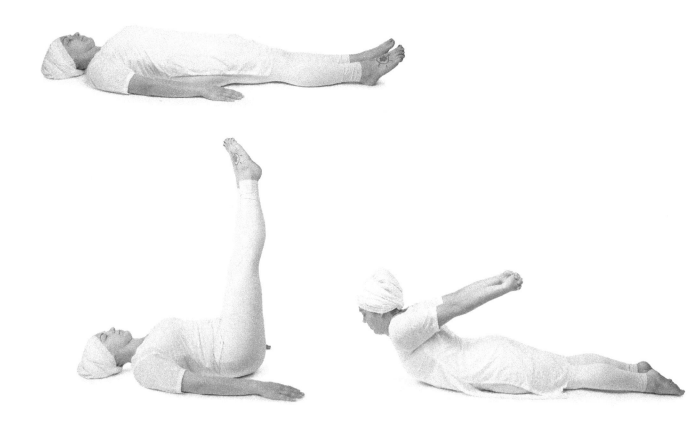

PART FOUR

Time: 1-3 Minutes

Lie on the back, arms at the sides, legs together. Inhale and raise both legs up to 90 degrees, knees straight, feet relaxed. Exhale and lower the legs. Breathe powerfully, creating a steady rhythm. Continue for 1-3 minutes.

PART FIVE

Time: 1-3 Minutes

Lie on the stomach, chin on the ground. Interlock the fingers in Venus Lock at the small of the back.

Inhale, raise the head and keeping the elbows straight stretch the arms up as far as possible. Close the eyes. Breathe Breath of Fire. Continue for 1-3 minutes.

To End: Inhale, exhale and relax.

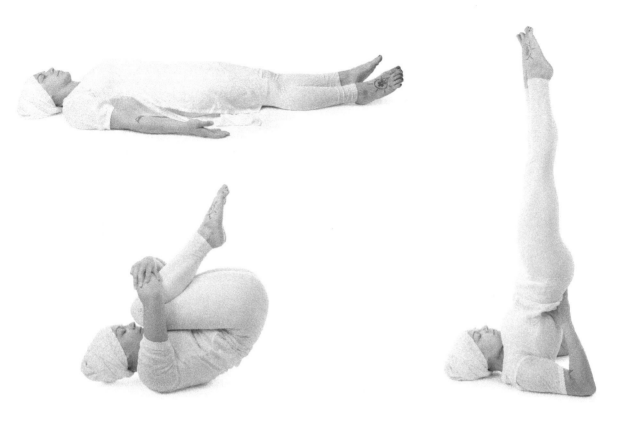

PART SIX

Time: 1-3 Minutes

Relax on the back the arms at the sides, palms face up.

After 1-3 minutes, bend the knees into the chest, wrap the arms around the legs, bringing the forehead toward the knees. Rock forward and back on the entire length of the spine. Continue for 1 minute.

PART SEVEN

Time: 1-3 Minutes

Lie on the back, place the hands on the back of the hips just below the waist. Inhale and lift the hips and legs up to a vertical position, the spine and legs perpendicular to the ground. Support the weight of the body on the elbows and shoulders use the hands to support the lower spine. Press the chin into the chest; Shoulder Stand. Breathe Breath of Fire. Continue for 1-3 minutes. Immediately begin Part Eight.

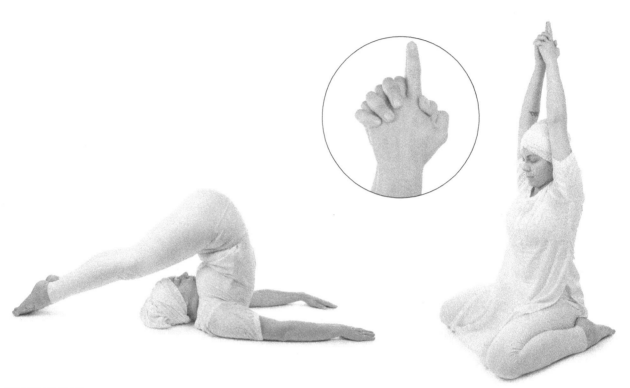

PART EIGHT

Time: 1-3 Minutes

Remain in Shoulder Stand, continue Breath of Fire, bend at the hips, carefully lower the feet to the ground behind the head, the knees are straight and toes pointed. Ideally, the back is straight and perpendicular to the ground. Keep the hands on the back for support or bring the arms to the ground pointing away from the body with interlaced the fingers; Plow Pose. With the breath slowly stretch the legs farther away from the torso, feel a mild stretch in the upper back and neck. Continue for 1-3 minutes.

To End: Inhale deeply. Exhale and relax the breath. Slowly come out of the posture. Support the back with the hands, bend the knees and release the spine to the ground, vertebra by vertebra, from the top of the spine to its base. Relax on the back.

PART NINE

Time: 3-5 Minutes

Sit between the heels with the feet on either side of the hips in Celibate Pose. Raise the hands above the head, palms together, interlace the fingers, extend the Jupiter Fingers (index fingers) straight up. For masculine energy cross the right thumb over the left, feminine cross left thumb over right.

Arms are straight and hug the ears. Chant SAT and powerfully draw the Navel Point in and up. Chant NAAM and release the Navel Point; Sat Kriya (in Celibate Pose). Continue for 3-5 minutes.

To End: Inhale, hold the breath and squeeze the muscles tightly from the buttocks all the way up the back. Mentally allow the energy to flow through the top of the skull. Exhale and relax.

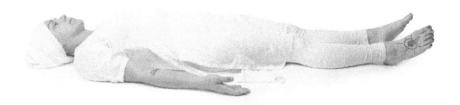

PART TEN

Time: 3-10 Minutes

Relax completely on the back for 3-10 minutes.

Comments: As human beings, we share certain instincts with animals, but we also have the ability to direct, shape and give meaning to the expression of these instincts. Many of the strongest instincts find expression and representation through the Lower Triangle of chakras, which include the First, Second and Third Chakras. The physical correlates of these chakras are the rectum, the sex organs and the Navel Point. Dysfunctions of the body are reflected in the mind and vice versa. A serious neurotic behavior or self-destructive attitude will also appear as an imbalance in the Lower Triangle. One of the most direct ways to correct such an imbalance is physically to stimulate the nervous and glandular systems in order to alter the instinctual and learned patterns in the lower chakras. Once this is achieved and a new energy balance is attained, then, through analytic self-assessment and meditation, it is possible to effect the holistic change in behavior, which is desired. This kriya is an example of such a technology. To use it correctly, remember to focus the mind on what you are doing and experiencing during this kriya.

Meditation Kriya for the Negative Mind

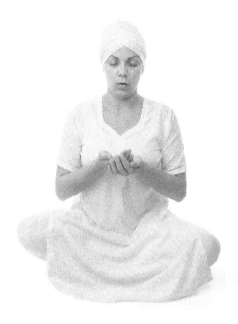

Time: 11 - 31 minutes

Sit in Easy Pose with a straight spine. Make a cup with both hands, palms face up, the right hand resting on the left hand. The fingers will cross. Bend the elbows, relaxed at the sides, place the hands at the level of the Heart Center. Eyes are slightly open and look down toward the hands. Inhale deeply in a long steady stroke through the nose. Exhale in a focused stream through rounded lips, feel the breath go over the hands. Let any thought or desire that is negative or persistently distracting come into the mind. Breathe the thought or feeling in, exhale it out with the breath. Continue for 11-31 minutes.

To End: Exhale completely and suspend the breath out, lock in the navel point. Concentrate on each vertebra of the spine until it feels stiff as a rod from top to bottom. Inhale powerfully, exhale completely, and repeat the mental concentration on the spine. Repeat the breath and concentration on the spine 3 to 5 times.

Comments: When you need to balance the flashing negativity and protective fervor of the Negative Mind, use this meditation. It clears the subconscious of unwanted negative or fearful thoughts. Then the Negative Mind can give you clear signals to protect and promote you. The posture is one of calmness and humility that lets the Creator, the Unknown, cover and shield you.

Kriya Set for Harnessing the Animal Force

August 1985

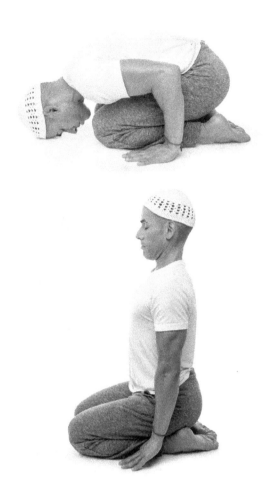

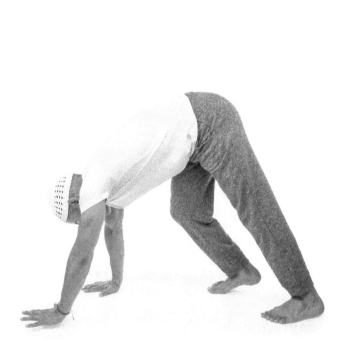

PART ONE

Time: 5 Minutes

Begin in Triangle Pose. Hands and feet on the ground, hips high, distribute the body's weight evenly on hands and feet, keep the arms and legs straight, create an equilateral triangle with the body. Walk in this position. Move very slowly forward, inch by inch. Continue for 5 minutes.

PART TWO

Time: 5 Minutes

Sit on the heels with a straight spine. Place the palms on the ground next to the legs. Exhale, bend forward, touch the forehead to the ground. Inhale, return to original position. Do not move the hands. Continue for 5 minutes.

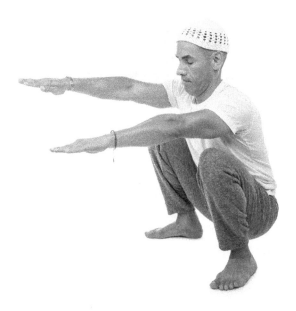

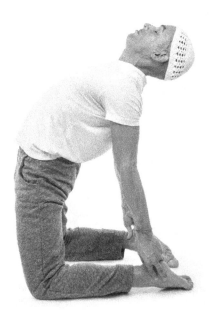

PART THREE

Time: 5 Minutes

Stand with the feet wide apart, squat, keep the spine straight and the heels on the ground; Crow Pose. Stretch the arms forward from the shoulders, parallel to the ground, elbows straight, palms face down. Move alternate arms up and down 6-10 inches, as one moves up the other moves down. Breathe Breath of Fire. Continue for 5 minutes.

PART FOUR

Time: 5 Minutes

Stand on the knees, hip width apart, reach the hands back to hold the heels, lift the hips as high as you can, keep the hips over the knees; Camel Pose. Relax the head back without compressing the neck. Breathe Breath of Fire. Continue for 5 minutes.

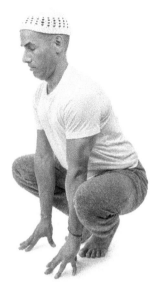

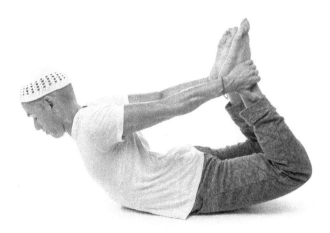

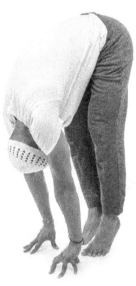

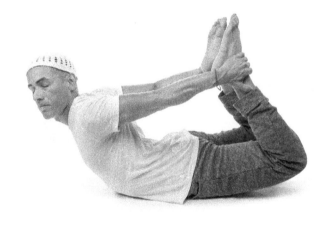

PART FIVE

Time: 5 Minutes

Stand with the heels together, toes apart. Squat, lift the heels off the ground and keep them together. Keep the knees wide, spine straight, head up; Frog Pose. Inhale, lift the hips, lower the head, keep the heels off the ground. Exhale, lower the hips to the original position. Continue for 5 minutes.

PART SIX

Time: 5 Minutes

Lie on the stomach, bend the knees and grasp the ankles. Lift the head, chest, knees and thighs off the ground, Bow Pose. Inhale, turn the head toward the right shoulder. Exhale, turn the head toward the left shoulder. Continue for 5 minutes.

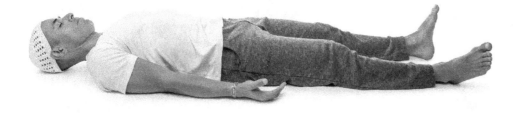

PART SEVEN

Time: 30 Minutes

Relax, continue to deepen the relaxation for 30 minutes.

Comments: These exercises will totally revitalize your entire body.

Meditation Kriya to Be Positive

February 10, 1998

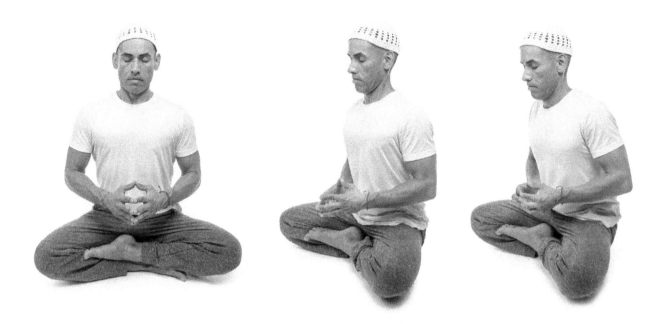

PART ONE

Sit in Easy Pose with a straight spine.

Mudra: With the elbows relaxed at the sides of the body, forearms parallel to the ground, place all fingertips together, fingers are straight and relaxed, keep space between them. Palms do not touch fingers point away from the body and the thumbs point up.

Movement: Keeping the fingertips touching and the fingers straight, bend the first knuckle at the junction of the hand and fingers and return. Simultaneously pull the lower spine forward, up, as the fingers open outward and relax the lower spine back as the knuckles bend. Keep the movement in the lower back. Move powerfully. Listen to Sat Naam Wahe Guru, Indian version #2 to keep the rhythm of the movement.

Eye position: Look at the Tip of the Nose.

Continue for 19 Minutes.

To End: Inhale and immediately begin Part 2.

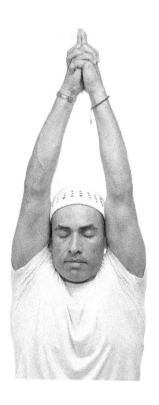

PART TWO

Movement: Continue the lower spinal motion. Raise the hands overhead, interlace the fingers and extend the Jupiter Fingers (index fingers) straight up, the elbows are straight. Moving powerfully, pull the body up. The music continues.

Eye position: Look at the Tip of the Nose.

Continue for 2 minutes.

To End: Inhale deep, hold the breath and stretch up, pull up with the hands to uplift the entire spine and body for 10 seconds. Cannon Fire exhale. Repeat 2 more times. Drop the hands in the lap with the last exhale.

Comments: In just a few minutes, this meditation changes your negative thoughts to positive. If for 40 days you can reduce your negative thoughts, you will totally change how to relate to others and show people how to be positive. This will change your life and others' lives.

Kriya For Glands, Circulation and Meditative Mind

November 9, 1983

Set A:

Time: 9-10 Minutes

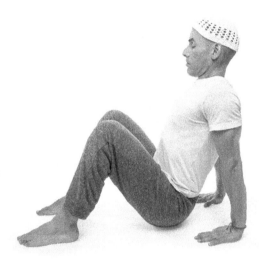

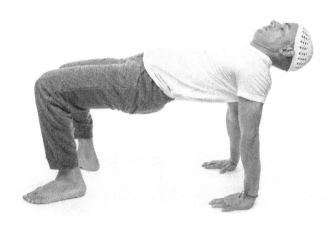

PART ONE

Time: 2 ¼ Minutes

Squat into Crow Pose. Place the palms flat on the ground behind the buttocks, arms straight, neck locked. Inhale, raise the hips up, spine parallel to the ground. Hold the posture and move the head up and down as fast as possible with Breath of Fire.

After 15 seconds, continue Breath of Fire, apply neck lock, lower and raise the hips rapidly and powerfully. Continue for 2 minutes.

Comments: This exercise works on the thyroid and parathyroid and adjusts the spine, glandular system and Navel Point.

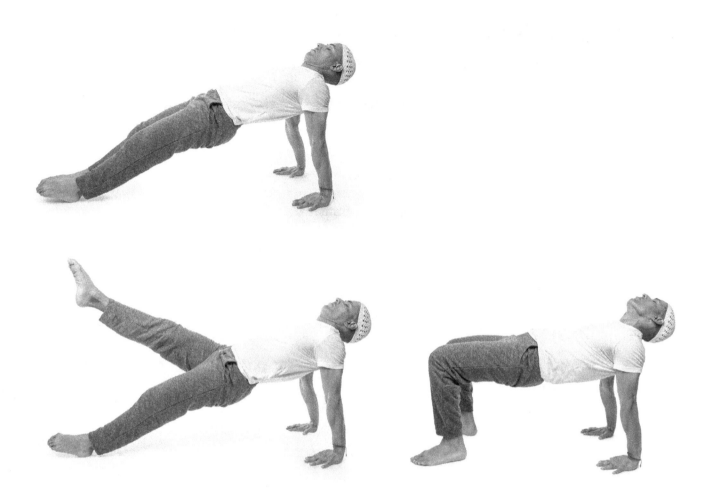

PART TWO

Time: 2 Minutes

Sit with the legs together, stretched straight forward. Place the palms flat on the ground behind the hips. Raise the hips up, create a straight line from the head to the toes; Back Platform Pose. Hold the posture, begin alternate leg lifts, raise the leg on the inhale, lower the leg on the exhale. Move quickly. Continue for 2 minutes.

PART THREE

Time: 1 Minute

Sit with the knees bent, feet flat on the ground. Place the palms flat on the ground behind the hips; fingers point forward, arms straight, apply neck lock. Raise the hips up, spine parallel to the ground; Bridge Pose. Hold the posture, inhale, rotate the head on the neck ½ way around, exhale powerfully, rotate the head the rest of the way around, use an explosive exhale to complete the rotation of the neck. Continue for 1 minute.

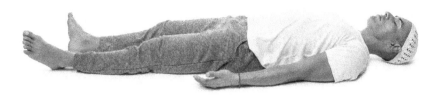

PART FOUR

Time: 4 ¾ Minutes

Relax on the back for 4 ¾ minutes.

Set B:

Time: 17 – 21 Minutes

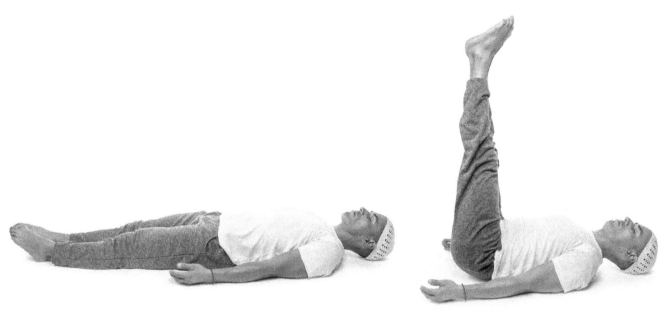

PART ONE

Time: 6 Minutes

Lie on the back. Point the toes, feet together, heels touch. Relax the hands at the sides of the body, palms face down. Consciously relax the body from the Navel Point up. Inhale, slowly raise the legs to 90 degrees, knees straight, legs close together, keep the toes pointed. Exhale, slowly lower the legs. Breathe slow, long and deep. Maintain the mental division of the body, totally relax from the Navel Point up. Continue for 6 minutes.

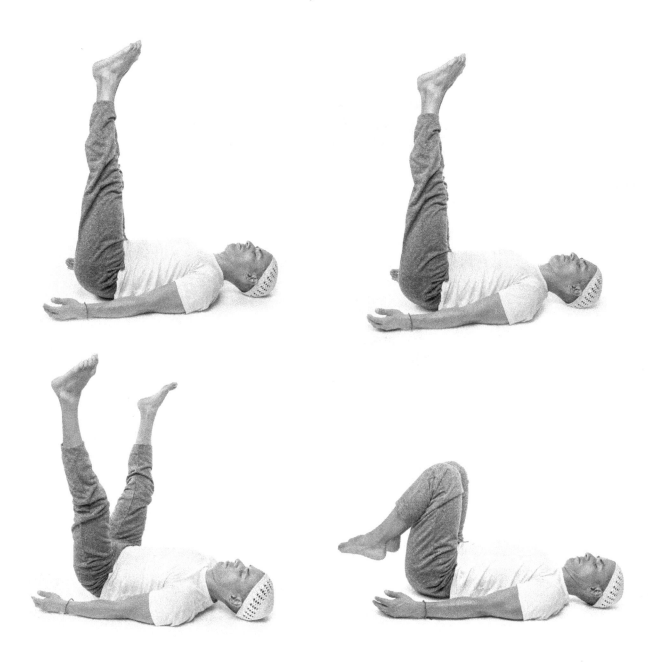

PART TWO

Time: 5 ½ Minutes

Remain on the back, arms at the sides, palms face down. Raise the legs together to 90 degrees, keep the knees straight, point the toes. Inhale, open the legs as wide as possible. Exhale, bring the legs back to 90 degrees. Continue for 5 ½ minutes.

PART THREE

Time: 1 ¾ Minutes

Remain on the back, arms at the sides, palms face down. Inhale, raise the legs together to 90 degrees. Exhale, quickly bend the knees and strike the buttocks forcefully with the heels. Continue at a very fast pace for 1 ¾ minutes.

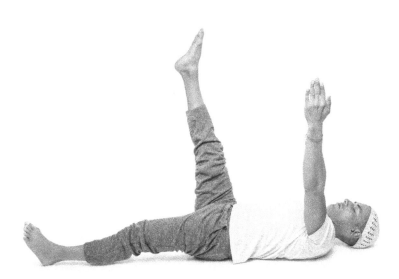
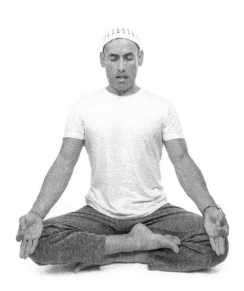

PART FOUR

Time: 1 ½ Minutes

Remain on the back, arms at the sides. Inhale raise the right leg and left arm up to 90 degrees. Exhale lower them. Keep the arm and leg straight. Alternate sides with a powerful breath;, move as fast as possible. Continue for 1 ½ minutes.

PART FIVE

Time: 4 Minutes

Sit in Easy Pose with a straight spine. Place the hands in Gyan Mudra on the knees. Chant HARA HARA HARA HARA HAREE HAR in monotone. The rhythm is as follows: 1 beat for each HARA HARA, 1 beat for HAREE (very short HA and held REE), 1 beat for HAR. Continue for 4 minutes.

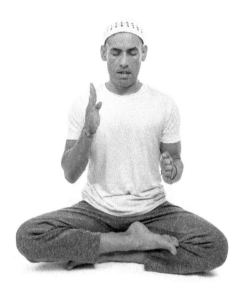

To End: Bend the elbows, bring the hands in front of the shoulders, palms face each other, fingers point up, hands relaxed. Move the hands opposite each other in small, extremely rapid forward and back movements. Chant HAR powerfully in monotone with the motion. Continue for 30 seconds. Inhale deep, hold the breath for 25 seconds. Exhale and relax.

Meditation Kriya for Tranquility and Peace

September 27, 1989

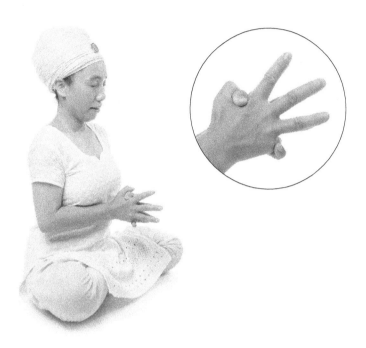

Instructions:

Eat a banana before practicing this kriya.

Sit in Easy Pose with a straight spine.

PART ONE

Time: 31 Minutes

Press the Jupiter Fingers (index fingers), Saturn Fingers (middle fingers) and Sun Fingers (ring fingers) together from the base of the fingers to the tips. Keep the pressed fingers straight and maintain a wide equal distance between the Jupiter Fingers, Saturn Fingers and Sun Fingers. They will want to come together. Cross the right thumb over the left and the right Mercury Finger (pinky finger) over the left, the base of the palms do not touch. The Saturn Fingers point straight forward at the level of the diaphragm. Press the elbows and forearms into the lower rib cage. Look at the Tip of the Nose and beyond to see the tip of the Jupiter Fingers. Lengthen the spine to the maximum and widen the shoulders. Take seven deep breaths to set the posture. Chant ONG NAMO GUROO DEV NAMO. *Ong Namo Guru Dev Namo* by Nirinjan Kaur was played in class. Continue for 31 minutes. Immediately begin Part Two.

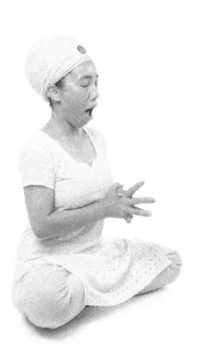 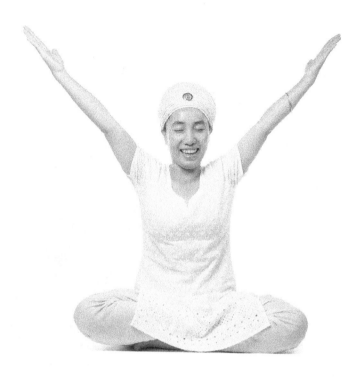

PART TWO

Time: 1.5 Minutes

Maintain the posture. Inhale deep, begin Breath of Fire, fast through a wide open mouth.

After 1 minute, inhale deep, close the mouth, breathe Breath of Fire powerfully from the navel. Continue for 30 seconds. Immediately begin Part Three.

PART THREE

Time: 1 minute

Remain in Easy Pose, inhale deep, raise the arms up to 60 degrees, hands relaxed, fingers together, thumbs relaxed, palms face each other, and laugh as loud as possible. Continue for 1 minute

To End: Inhale deep, hold the breath for 25 seconds and tighten the body as much as possible, open the fingers wide, palms face forward, contract all the muscles. Exhale. Repeat 2 more times. Relax.

Kriya for Physical and Mental Vitality

Spring 1970

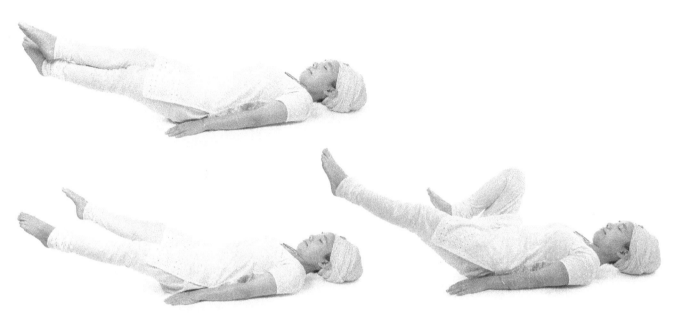

PART ONE

Time: 15 Minutes

Lie on your back and lift the legs to 12 inches. Spread the legs wide and crisscross left over right, then right over left. Keep the legs straight. Arms at the sides.

After 5 minutes, Inhale and apply *Mul Bandh*. Relax for 2 ½ minutes. Repeat the cycle.

PART TWO

Time: 15 Minutes

Lift both legs 2 feet off the ground. Begin a push-pull movement with the legs, bringing one knee in as the opposite leg is straight; keep the legs parallel to the ground. Relax the arms at the sides, palms down.

After 5 minutes, rest for 2 ½ minutes. Repeat the cycle.

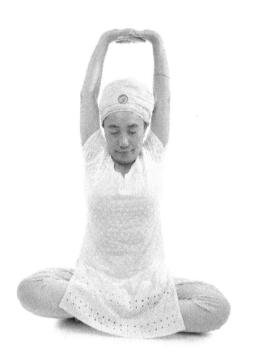

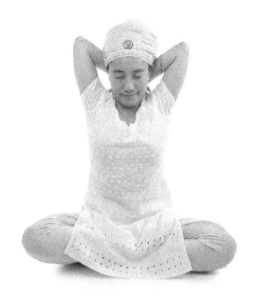

PART THREE

Time: 5 Minutes

Sit in Easy Pose with a straight spine. Lift
the arms straight above the head. Interlock
the fingers, turn the palms to face the sky.
Breathe Breath of Fire. Continue for 5
minutes. Feel the worries of the day fall away.
Feel the body rising above the clouds and
filled with the light energy of breath.

PART FOUR

Time: 5 Minutes

Remain in Easy Pose. Cross the arms behind
the head, grasping opposite shoulders with
the thumbs in front. Breathe Breath of Fire.
Continue for 5 minutes. Feel the light energy
lift into the head and project the mind into an
expansive peacefulness.

To End: Inhale, exhale, inhale, hold and circulate
the energy. Exhale and apply *Mul Bandh*.

Inhale, exhale, and apply *Mul Bandh* two
more times.

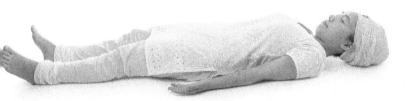

PART FIVE

Time: 5 Minutes

Lie on the back, relax completely. Separate the mental body from the physical body and move it around. Continue for 5 minutes. Come back into the physical body. Immediately begin Part Six.

PART SIX

Time is unspecified.

Sit in Easy Pose. Chant any divine mantra. Meditate.

Comments: This is a challenging kriya. When first practicing consider proportionately reducing the times of each part. The kriya moves the kundalini energy from the lower three chakras in Exercises 1, and 2; through the Heart Center in Exercise 3; and through the Throat Chakra to the higher centers in Exercise 4. The hard work automatically brings deep relaxation and meditation.

Meditation to Achieve Your Vastness

September 10, 1992

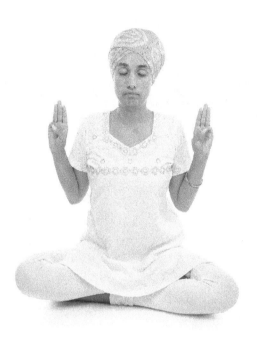

Instructions:

Sit in Easy Pose with a straight spine.

PART ONE

Time: 15 Minutes

Bend the elbows, relaxed at the sides. Hands are at the level of the shoulders, palms face forward in Buddhi Mudra (Thumb tips and Mercury Finger tips touch), the rest of the fingers are straight, together and point up. Eyes are 1/10th open and look at the Tip of the Nose. Inhale through the nose, exhale through the mouth, long and deep. Breathe consciously. Sit in a very peaceful, tranquil way. Continue for 15 minutes.

To End: Inhale deep, hold the breath for 15 seconds. Cannon Fire exhale. Repeat two more times. Relax.

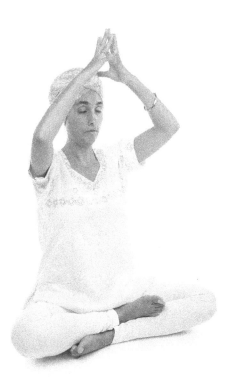

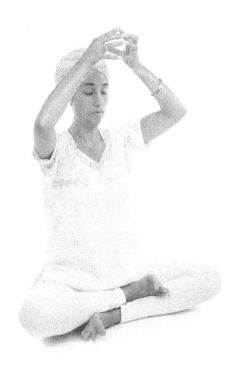

PART TWO

Time: 11 Minutes

Remain in Easy Pose. Raise the arms, bend the elbows, hands are above and in front of the forehead within the arc line. Place all five finger tips together, palms do not touch. Keep the finger tips together while moving the fingers in circles, the wrists will move. Simultaneously move all of the toes. Create a rhythm. Continue for 11 minutes, move the fingers and toes faster and harder for the last 1 ½ minutes.

To End: Inhale deep, hold the breath for 15 seconds, move fast. Cannon Fire exhale through the mouth. Repeat two more times. Relax.

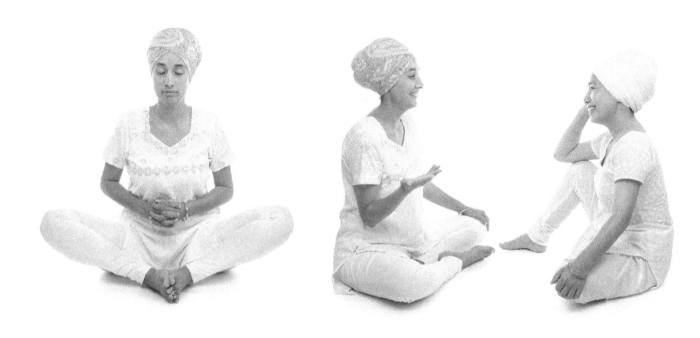

PART THREE

Time: 9 ½ Minutes

Sit with a straight spine and bring the soles of the feet together. Interlace the fingers, hold them tight. Place the hands in front of the solar plexus. Move the shoulders in large forward circles. Continue for 9 ½ minutes.

To End: Inhale deep, hold the breath for 15 seconds, move the shoulders. Cannon Fire exhale. Repeat two more times. Relax and talk to each other; have fun.

Kriya for Balancing the Three Psyches

May 24, 1984

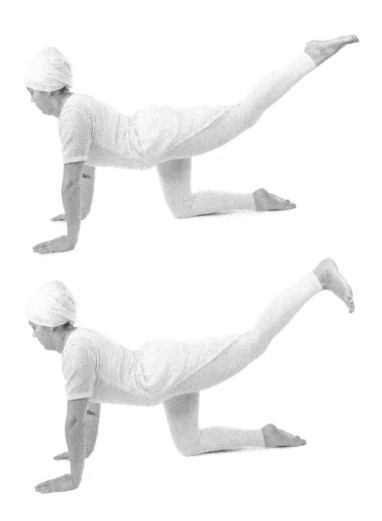

PART ONE

Time: 4 ½ Minutes

Come onto the hands and knees in Cow Pose. Extend the left leg back and raise it to sixty degrees. Point and flex the left foot in rhythm with a powerful Breath of Fire.

The breath and the foot must move at the same speed.

After 3 minutes, Switch legs and continue for 1 ½ minutes. Immediately begin Part Two.

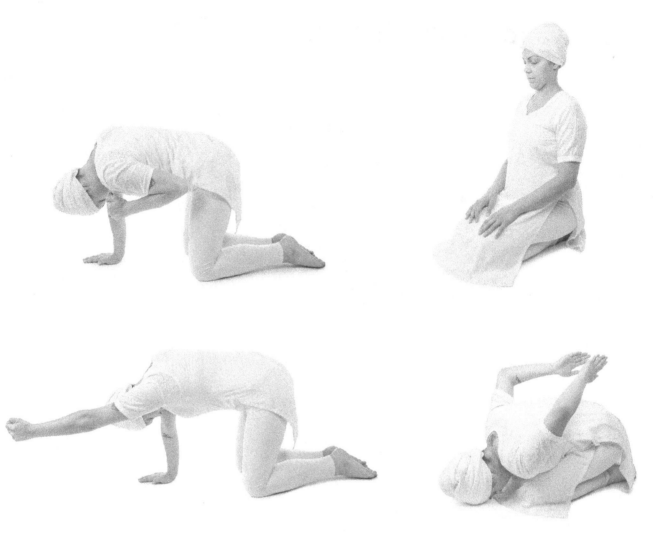

PART TWO

Time: 3 ½ Minutes

Remain on the hands and knees, move into Cat Pose. Make a fist with the left hand in front of the Heart Center. Strongly punch the fist forward and back in rhythm with Breath of Fire. The hand and arm are as tough as steel and the breath is rhythmic and powerful. The shoulder blade must move.

After 2 minutes, Switch arms and continue for 1 ½ minutes. Immediately begin Part Three.

PART THREE

Time: 3 ½ Minutes

Sit on the heels with a straight spine, Rock Pose. Bow and touch the forehead to the floor, simultaneously powerfully clap the hands behind the back. Return to the starting position. Continue the movement for 3 ½ minutes. Immediately begin Part Four.

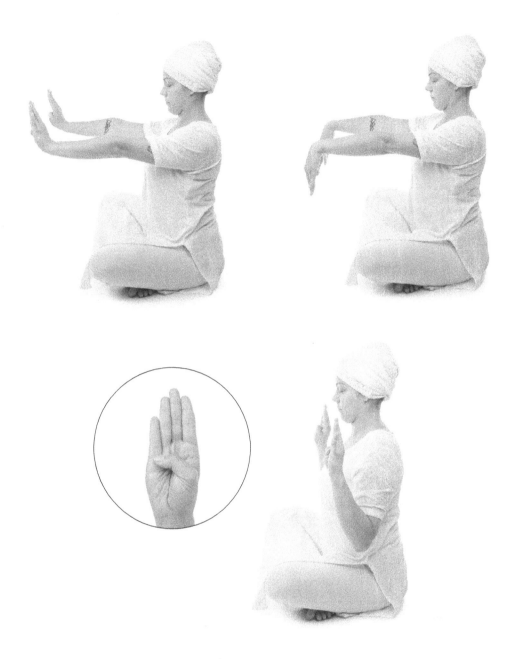

PART FOUR

Time: 1 ½ Minutes

Sit in Easy Pose with a straight spine. Bring the arms out straight forward parallel to the ground, palms face down. Touch the thumbs to the mounds at the base of the Mercury Fingers (pinky fingers). Move the hands rapidly up and down at the wrist eight times. (These eight movements take about 2 seconds). Immediately bend the elbows, rapidly pull the arms back, the elbows hit the rib cage, the forearms are perpendicular to the ground, palms face forward. The motion takes 1 second. Extend your arms and repeat the eight count hand movement. Continue the sequence for 1 ½ minutes. Immediately begin Part Five.

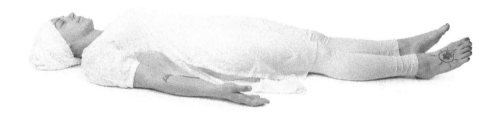

PART FIVE

Time: 5 – 11 Minutes

Lie down on the back. Relax completely for 5-11 minutes. (The gong was played in class, concentrate at the Heart Center on the beat of the heart.)

To End: Move the neck, slowly and powerfully roll the neck and slowly sit up in Easy Pose. Roll your shoulders and hips and relax.

Comments: Projectivity in Kundalini Yoga balances the intelligence. Sometimes the psyche of intelligence is not balanced with the psyche around you. There are three psyches: your individual inner psyche, the psyche which is in your immediate environment, and the psyche of the landscape which is bigger, higher, and wider. If these three psyches are not in balance, you are not in harmony.

The problem with you is that you think money, relationships and power can make you harmonious, but if your own psyche is not in harmony, nothing can make you harmonious.

Meditation Kriya to Time Yourself

September 27, 1989

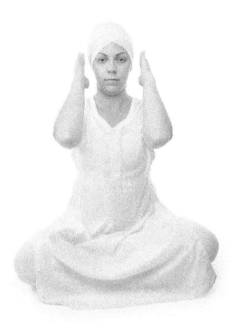
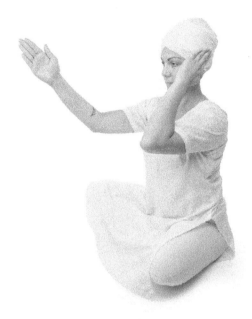

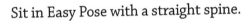

Sit in Easy Pose with a straight spine.

Posture: Bend the elbows and bring the hands on either side of the ears, fingers straight and together, thumbs relaxed. Hands are tense with palms facing the head. Move one forearm and hand approximately 12 inches forward from the ear, while the other forearm and hand moves back to the ear. Move from the elbows at a fast, comfortable pace, 1 cycle per second.

Eye position: Look straight. Keep looking straight for 1 minute, then slowly and gradually close the eyes and roll them down to look at the Moon Center (chin).

Mantra: Listen to *Har, Har, Gobinday* by Nirinjan Kaur, the Prosperity Mantra.

Continue for 22 minutes.

To End: Music ends. Inhale deep, hold it, hold the hands steady by the ears with a straight spine for 25 seconds. Exhale through the mouth. Repeat 2 more times and relax.

Kriya for Auric Balance and Nerve Strength

April 7, 1974

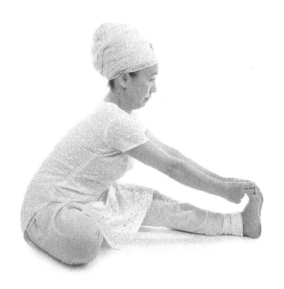

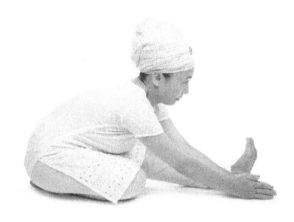

PART ONE

Time: 3-5 Minutes

Sit with the left leg straight forward. Bring the heel of the right foot next to the groin with sole against the inner thigh. Lean forward from the hips, spine straight. Lock the first two fingers of both hands around the big toe, press the toenail with the thumbs. Lift the chin, look above the horizon. Breathe in the following sequence: Inhale in four parts, mentally chant SAA, TAA, NAA, MAA. Hold the breath for sixteen parts, mentally chant the mantra four times. Exhale in two parts, mentally chant WHAA HAY GUROO. Continue for 3-5 minutes. The breath is the key to this kriya.

PART TWO

Time: 3-5 Minutes

Remain seated with the left leg straight forward. Bend the right knee and sit on the right heel. Lean forward from the hips. Place the palms together, fingers straight, Prayer Pose. Stretch the arms straight forward on the ground. Lift the chin, look above the horizon. Breathe in the same sequence as Part One. Continue for 3-5 minutes.

To End: Inhale and relax for 1 minute.

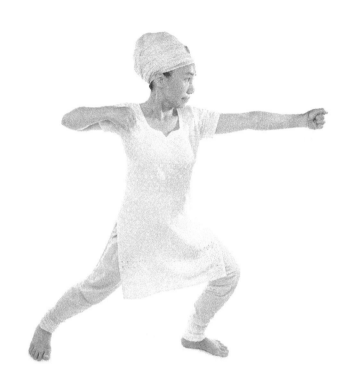

PART THREE

Time: 3-5 Minutes

Stand up, come into Archer Pose with the left leg forward. Gaze over the extended fist to the horizon. Breathe in the same sequence as Part One. Continue for 3-5 minutes.

To End: Inhale and relax into meditation.

Comments: This set is a jewel. It has been used to initiate students into the deeper "mysteries" and effects of Kundalini Yoga. It develops your nerve strength and aura. After practicing this set, meditate for as long as you like. This set stimulates the basic evolutionary power of your consciousness. In difficult times, it will enable you to help others.

Meditation for a Powerful Protective Aura

September 12, 1989

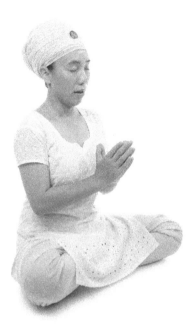

Time: 22 Minutes

Sit in Easy Pose with a straight spine. Relax the arms at the sides of the body. Bend the elbows. Bring the hands together in front of the Heart Center. Press the hands together, thumbs extended back towards the body. Angle the hands 45 degrees away from the body. Apply just enough pressure to keep the hands together. Look at the tips of the thumbs. Chant the following mantra in a monotone:

GUROO GUROO WHAA – HAY GUROO GUROO RAAM DAAS GUROO.

Each sound is clipped short except WHAA which is not clipped. Repeat the mantra 3 times on each breath.

After 11 minutes, inhale deeply and exhale completely three times. Repeat the meditation for another 11 minutes.

To End: Inhale deeply and exhale completely five times.

Comments: This mudra held at the center of the chest balances the flow of energy. The meditation builds the protection and power of the aura.

Kriya for the Lymph Glands

October 26, 1983

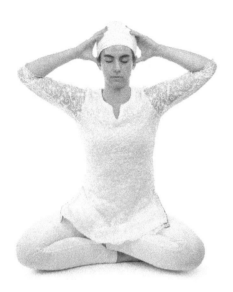
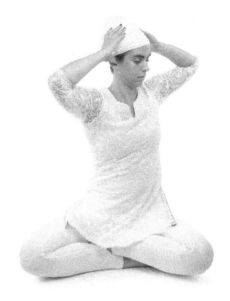

PART ONE

Time: 3 Minutes

Sit in Easy Pose with a straight spine. Place the fingers on top of the head, the thumbs completely closing off the ears, elbows out to the sides. Twist left, return to center, twist right, return to center, each movement is separate. The breath is not specified. Continue for 3 minutes. Immediately begin Part Two.

Mastery of the True Self

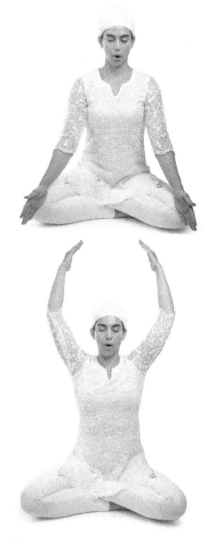

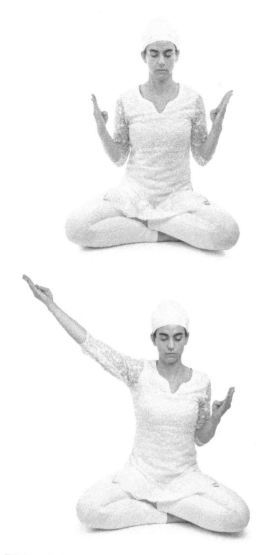

PART TWO

Time: 3-4 Minutes

Remain in Easy Pose. Press the thumbs on the Mercury Mounds (just beneath the pinkie fingers).

Bend the elbows, relaxed by the sides and bring the hands near the shoulders, palms face the body.

Apply Neck Lock, with chin in and chest out throughout the exercise. Raise one arm up to 60 degrees, reverse, as one hand goes up the other goes down in a fast powerful push-pull motion. Keep the palms facing in. Move with the breath, it becomes like a powerful Breath of Fire. Continue for 3-4 minutes. Immediately begin Part Three.

PART THREE

Time: 4-5 Minutes

Remain in Easy Pose, place the hands on the knees, palms facing up. The hands are relaxed but firm.

Inhale with the mouth open wide, lips rounded, making a deep heavy sound with the breath. With the inhale lift the arms high up and back over the head, elbows bend slightly. Exhale through the mouth, return the hands to the knees. This exercise is done powerfully and as the movement continues, the hands may not reach the knees. As the exercise continues, this sound will become like a lion's roar. Continue for 4-5 minutes. Immediately begin Part Four.

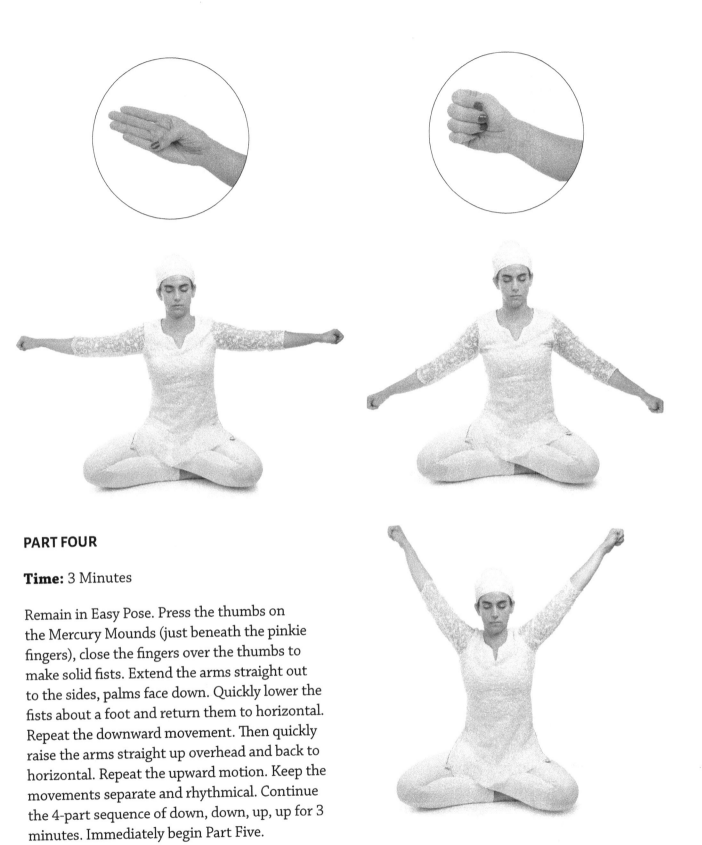

PART FOUR

Time: 3 Minutes

Remain in Easy Pose. Press the thumbs on the Mercury Mounds (just beneath the pinkie fingers), close the fingers over the thumbs to make solid fists. Extend the arms straight out to the sides, palms face down. Quickly lower the fists about a foot and return them to horizontal. Repeat the downward movement. Then quickly raise the arms straight up overhead and back to horizontal. Repeat the upward motion. Keep the movements separate and rhythmical. Continue the 4-part sequence of down, down, up, up for 3 minutes. Immediately begin Part Five.

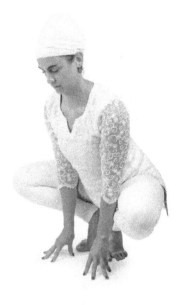

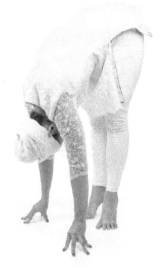

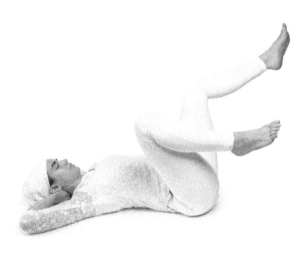

PART FIVE

108-240 Repetitions

Squat down in Frog Pose, on the toes, heels together and off the ground, knees wide. Place the fingertips on the ground between the knees. The face is forward. Inhale, raise the hips up, keep the fingertips on the ground and the heels off the ground. Exhale, return to original position. Breathe powerfully and move rapidly. Continue for 3 to 4 minutes. Immediately begin Part Six.

PART SIX

Time: 3 Minutes

Lie down on the back. Place the hands in Venus Lock under the neck. Bring the legs up and begin a bicycling motion, as if you were riding a bicycle in the air. Move the feet in big circles (not a push-pull movement). Continue for 3 minutes. Immediately begin Part Seven.

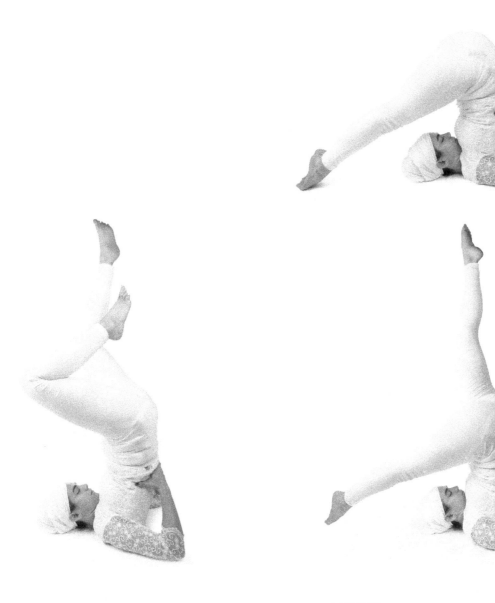

PART SEVEN

Time: 2-3 Minutes

Lie on the back, place the hands on the back of the hips, just below the waist. Bring the hips up high, spine and legs perpendicular to the ground. Support the weight of the body on the elbows and shoulders. Use the hands to support the lower spine, press the chin into the chest, Shoulder Stand. Begin a bicycling motion, move the feet in big circles. Continue for 2-3 minutes. Immediately begin Part Eight.

PART EIGHT

Time: 1 Minute

Remain in Shoulder Stand. Lower the legs down over the head, toes touch the ground, legs are straight, Plow Pose. Raise the legs alternately in a scissor motion. Move quickly and powerfully. Continue for 1 minute.

To End: Gently lower the knees toward the head, release the spine to the ground vertebrae by vertebrae.

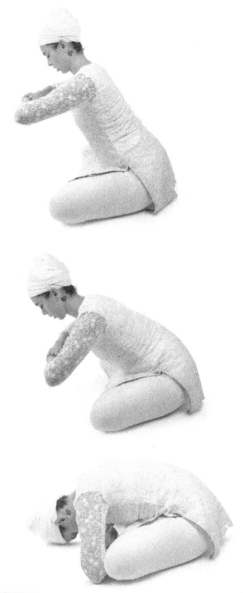

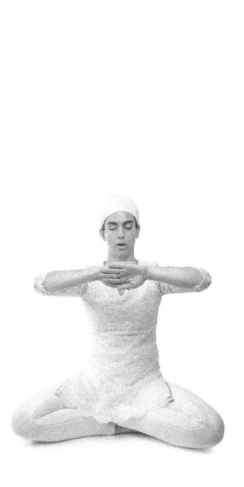

PART NINE

Time: 1 Minute

Sit in Easy Pose with a straight spine. Raise the arms to shoulder level, bend the elbows and bring the left hand in front of the right. Palms face forward. Right palm touches the back of the left hand. Chant the mantra: HAR GUROO SIREE GUROO WAA-HAY GUROO in monotone. One repetition takes 6 seconds. Continue for 1 minute. Immediately begin Part Ten.

PART TEN

Time: 5-6 Minutes

Maintain the posture. Use the same chant: Bend forward from the hips one third of the way down as HAR GUROO is chanted. Move two-thirds of the way down with SIREE GUROO. Touch the hands and head to the ground with WAA-HAY GUROO (maintain the mudra.) Come up very quickly, and continue without breaking the rhythm for 5-6 minutes. Immediately begin Part Eleven.

PART ELEVEN

Time: 1-3 Minutes

Maintain the posture, bend forward with the arms and forehead touching the ground. Breathe a heavy Breath of Fire.

After 1 minute, relax the breath and rest in this posture for 1 to 3 minutes as you say your own silent prayer.

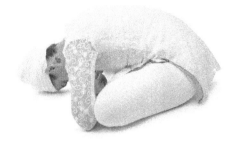

Comments: When the lymph glands aren't doing their job, and the lungs aren't working properly, dead cells and mucous in the lungs do not clear out. If this continues, ultimately you could get seriously ill.

Praanic Kriya to Build Vitality

December 4, 1991

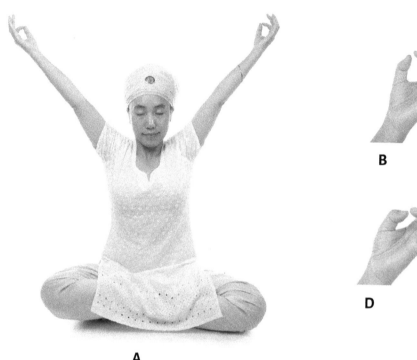

A

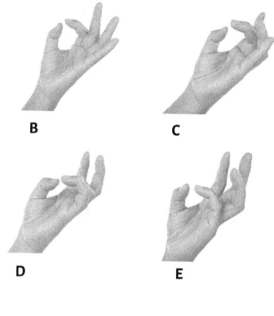

This set requires a banana and an orange.

Sit in Easy Pose with a straight spine.

PART ONE

Time: 14 Minutes

Raise the arms up and out to 60 degrees, elbows straight. Quickly tap the thumb tips and Jupiter Finger (index finger) tips together, the rest of the fingers are relaxed, keep the wrists straight, palms face up. Look at the Tip of the Nose.

After 9 minutes, change to tapping the thumb tips and Saturn Fingers (middle fingers).

After 1 minute, change to tapping the thumb tips and Sun Fingers (ring fingers).

After 1 minute, change to tapping the thumb tips and Mercury Fingers (pinky fingers). Continue for 3 minutes.

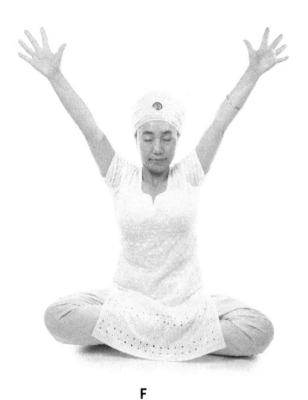

F

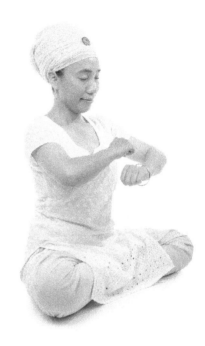

PART TWO

To End: Maintain the posture. Palms forward, open the fingers wide, straight and tense. Breathe heavy Breath of Fire for 30 seconds. Inhale deep, suspend the breath for 10 seconds, tighten the body. Cannon Fire exhale. Inhale deep, suspend the breath for 15 seconds, tighten every part of the body. Cannon Fire exhale. Inhale deep, inhale a little more, suspend the breath for 25 seconds, lift and open the rib cage, tighten the body. Cannon Fire exhale. Relax for 1 minute.

Time: 1.5 Minutes

Remain in Easy Pose with a straight spine. Press the thumbs into the Mercury Mound (just under the pinky fingers), lock the rest of the fingers tight over the thumbs. Rotate the fists palms down around each other in small outward circles at the Heart Center. Move fast. Continue for 1.5 minutes. Immediately begin Part Three.

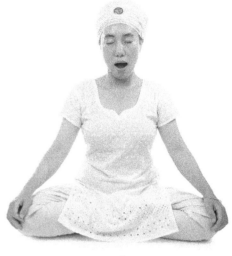

A

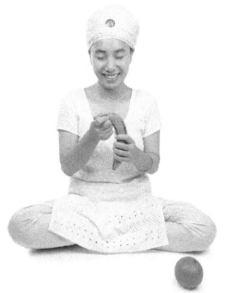

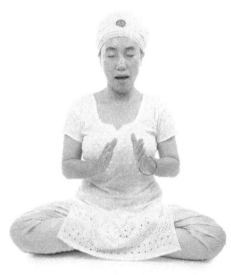

B

PART THREE

Time: 8 Minutes

Remain in Easy Pose. Close the eyes. Peel and eat the banana and orange without opening the eyes. Continue for 8 minutes. Immediately begin Part Four.

PART FOUR

Time: 2.5 Minutes

Remain in Easy Pose with a straight spine. Keep the eyes closed. Tighten the lips together and "pop" them open to create a sound with the mouth and lips. Make noise, 2 "pops" per second.

After 2 minutes, clap the hands with the sound. Continue for 30 seconds.

To End: Relax. Open the eyes and look at each other for 30 seconds. Immediately begin Part Five.

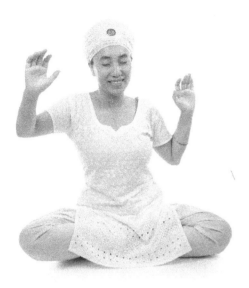

PART FIVE

Time: 10 Minutes

Remain in Easy Pose. Play *Punjabi Drums* and
dance the body. Move the shoulders, arms, hands
and rib cage. Continue for 10 minutes. Relax.
Drink a lot of water after practicing this kriya.

Kriya Guardian of Health

July 4, 1985

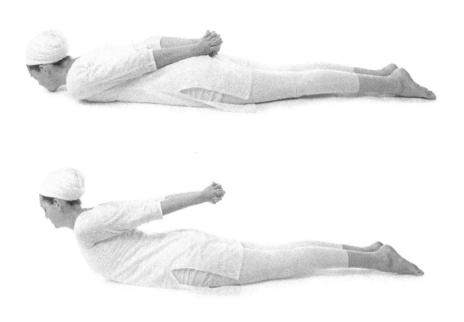

PART ONE

Time: 6 Minutes

Lie on the stomach. Place the chin on the ground, interlock the hands behind the back. Inhale, raise the head, chest and arms as high as possible. Keep the legs on the ground. Exhale, relax down to original position. Continue rhythmically inhaling up and exhaling down for 6 minutes.

Comments: This posture helps maintain the health of the lymphatic system.

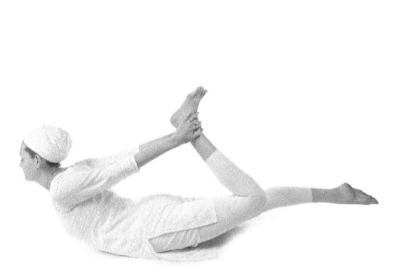

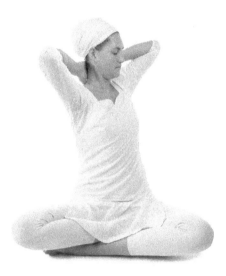

PART TWO

Time: 8 Minutes

Remain on the stomach. Bend the left knee, grasp the ankle with both hands. Inhale, lift the head, chest and leg as high as possible. Exhale, relax to original position. Continue the movement for 6 minutes. Switch ankles and continue for 2 more minutes.

Comments: This posture stretches the ovaries and helps regulate the menstrual cycle. It also tones your back muscles and maintains the elasticity of your spine, improving posture and increasing vitality.

PART THREE

Time: 2 Minutes

Sit in Easy Pose with a straight spine. Interlock the hands behind the neck at the hairline. Keep the elbows wide, forearms parallel to the ground. Twist the torso left and right rhythmically with Breath of Fire. Continue for 2 minutes.

In this posture, the digestive tract is massaged releasing stored tension and adjusting the ovaries and fallopian tubes.

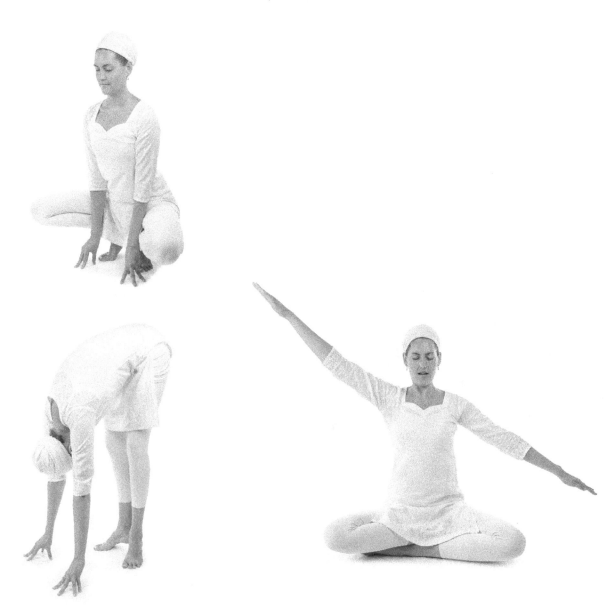

PART FOUR

108 Repetitions

Squat down with the heels together lifted off the ground. With the knees wide, place the fingertips on the ground in front of the feet, keeping the spine straight, head up, Frog Pose. Inhale, remain on the toes, and bring the forehead toward the knees. Exhale, return to the original position. Repeat the cycle 108 times.

PART FIVE

Time: 3 Minutes

Sit in Easy Pose with a straight spine. Extend the arms out to the sides parallel to the ground, palms face down. In a seesaw motion, raise the right arm up 60 degrees while lowering the left arm down 60 degrees, keep the wrists straight. Continue this motion, counting 1 to 12, on 13, clap the hands over the head. Continue this sequence.

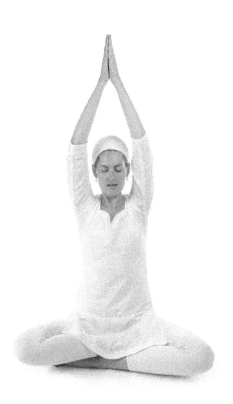

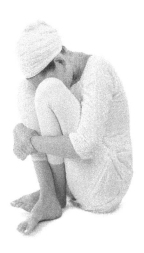

After 1 minute, replace the counting with the mantra HAREE HAR (HAREE is 1, HAR is 2). Repeat the mantra 6 times. Chant FATEH and clap the hands over the head. Continue for 2 minutes.

PART SIX

Time: 8 Minutes

Remain in Easy Pose. Bring the knees up and together, keep the ankles crossed. Wrap the arms around the shins, clasp the left wrist with the right hand. Rest the forehead on the knees. Breathe long and deep. Relax completely into the posture. Continue for 8 minutes. (Musical variation: Sing with *Mulh Mantra* by Singh Kaur for 4 minutes. Switch music to *Ardaas Bhaee* by Singh Kaur. Sing along for 4 minutes.)

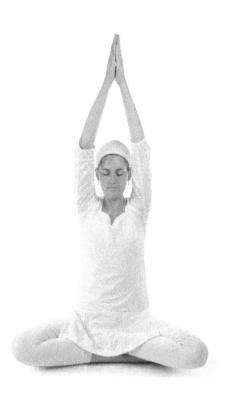

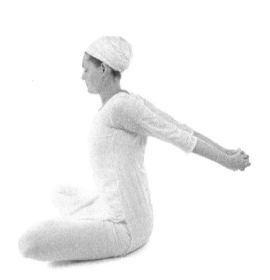

PART SEVEN

Time: 9 Minutes

Sit in Easy Pose with a straight spine. Breathe steady, long, deep and meditatively. Assume the following postures for 1 minute each, assess their different effects (Musical variation: Sing with *Ardaas Bhaee* by Singh Kaur throughout the postures.):

Raise the arms high over the head, palms together.

Interlock the fingers at the base of the spine, lift the arms away from the back as far as possible.

With the fingers interlocked, bend forward, bring the forehead to the ground and raise the arms as high as possible.

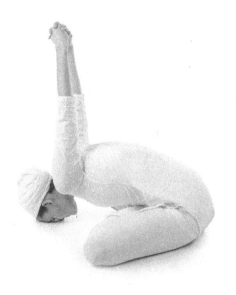

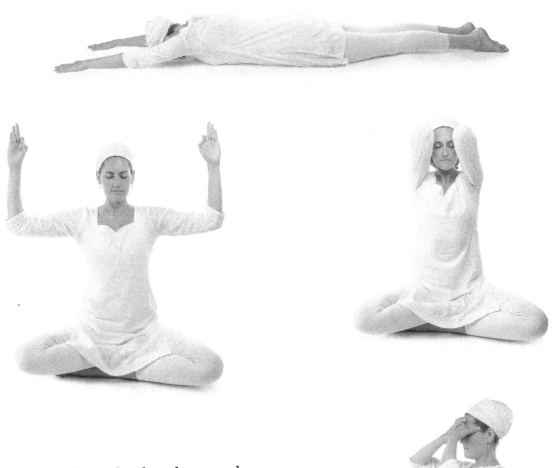

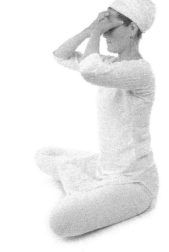

Lie on the stomach, forehead on the ground. Extend the arms forward on the ground, palms face down. Keep the legs straight and relaxed, tops of the feet are on the ground, Salutation to the Earth Posture.

Sit in Easy Pose with a straight spine. Extend the arms out to the sides, parallel to the ground, bend the elbows so the forearms are perpendicular to the ground, palms face forward, hands in Gyan Mudra.

Remain in Easy Pose. Interlock the fingers behind the neck at the hairline. Point the elbows forward. Press the forearms against the ears to block out any sound.

Remain in Easy Pose. Place the fingers flat on the forehead, right hand over left. Keep the fingers together, press the thumbs against the temples.

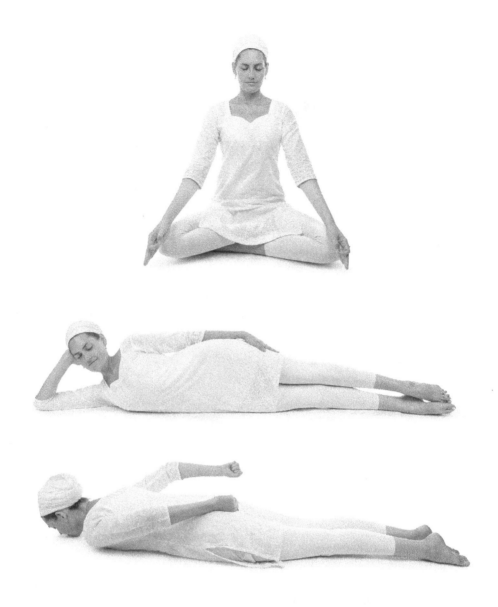

Remain in Easy Pose. Place the hands in Gyan Mudra on the knees, arms straight.

Lie down on the right side. Keep the body straight as an arrow, rest the head in the right palm. Rest the left arm on the left side of the body.

PART EIGHT

Time: 1 Minute

Lie on the stomach. Pound the buttocks with alternate fists. Continue for 1 minute.

This posture is outstanding for its simplicity and relaxing effects.

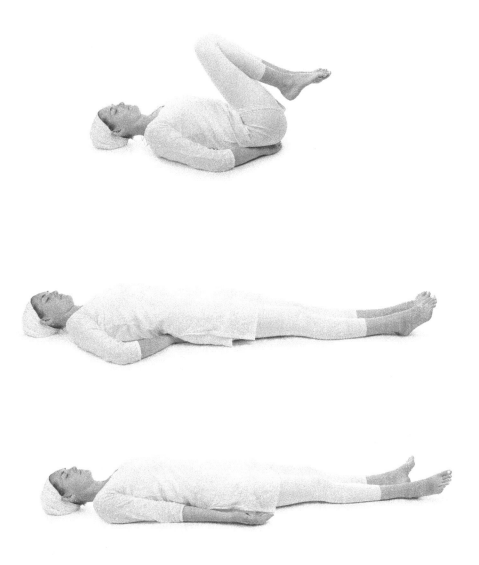

PART NINE

7 Minutes

Lie on the back. Place the hands under the small of the back, palms face down. Inhale, bring both knees to the chest. Exhale, keep the heels together and extend the legs straight onto the ground. Breathe powerfully. Keep a moderate steady pace. Continue for 7 minutes. (Musical variation: Chant HAR HAR MUNKANDE by Singh Kaur. Draw the knees into the chest on HAR HAR. Extend the legs straight on MUKANDE.)

PART TEN

Time not specified

Remain on the back, arms by the sides, palms face up. Relax completely. Listen to beautiful music.

Trataka Mudra Meditation

November 29, 1990

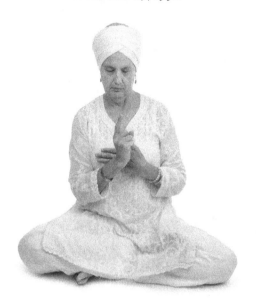

Sit in Easy Pose with a straight spine.

Mudra: Place the left hand on the Heart Center, fingers together pointing right, parallel to the ground, elbow relaxed. Bring the base of the right hand in front of the Heart Center. Extend the Jupiter Finger (index finger) straight up, hold the rest of the fingers down with the thumb, palm faces left.

Eyes: Look at the Tip of the Nose and at the tip of the Jupiter Finger. Align the tip of the finger with the Tip of the Nose to create one line of sight.

Mantra: Chant

ONG NAMO GUROO DEV NAMO.

Musical version by Nirinjan Kaur was played during class

Continue for **31 minutes**.

To End: Inhale deep, hold the breath tight and concentrate for 15 seconds. Exhale. Inhale deep, hold the breath tight and concentrate for 20 seconds. Exhale. Inhale deep, hold the breath tight and concentrate for 25 seconds. Exhale and relax. Talk to each other for 3 minutes.

Comment: This meditation will invoke in you the power to be intuitive so you can protect yourself.

Total Balance Kriya

October 26, 1983

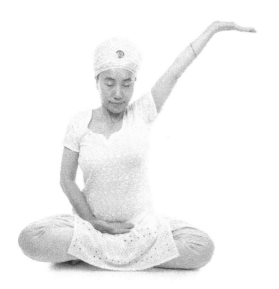 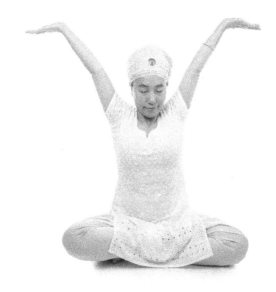

PART ONE

Time: 12 Minutes

Sit in Easy Pose with a straight spine. Rest the right hand in the lap, palm up. Lift the left arm up to the side at a 60-degree angle, palm face up, fingers together, extend the wrist and pull the fingers downward. Keep the elbow and spine straight. Stretch the palm and extend the wrist as much as possible; it will put pressure on the elbow.

After 4 minutes, switch arms, continue.

After 4 minutes, raise both arms into the same posture, sit calmly and let the energy balance. The breath will adjust itself. Continue for 4 minutes.

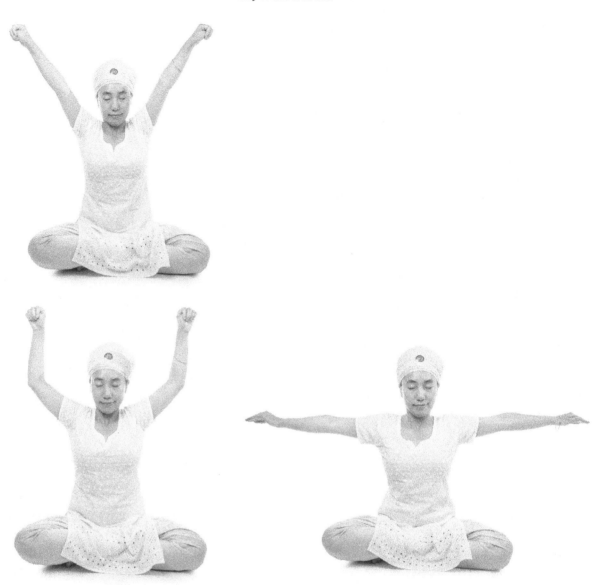

PART TWO

Time: 6 Minutes

Remain in Easy Pose. Raise the arms up to 60 degrees, make fists, place the thumbs inside the fists. Move the fists in slow circles on the wrists, direction not specified. Keep the elbows straight. Breath is not specified.

After 3 minutes, keep the hands in fists, bring the arms out parallel to the ground. Continue to circle the fists. Additionally, begin to circle the forearms from the elbows. Continue for 3 minutes.

PART THREE

Time: 10 Minutes

Remain in Easy Pose. Extend the arms out to side parallel to the ground, elbows straight. The head and neck are relaxed. Fingers and thumbs together, cup the hands slightly. Allow the breath to find its own pattern. DO not use Breath of Fire or heavy breathing. Continue for 10 minutes.

Comments: If you go past the stage of wanting to yell, there will come a time when Ahhh will just come out.

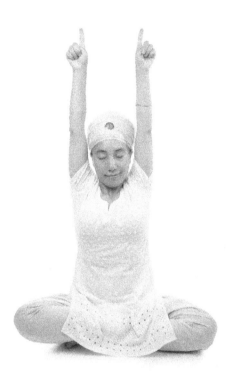

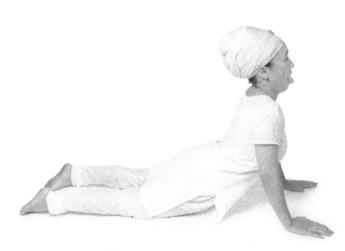

PART FOUR

Time: 2 Minutes

Remain in Easy Pose. Stretch the arms up over the head, elbows touch the ears. Make fists with the thumbs inside. One by one, stretch each finger and close it; first finger, close it; second finger, close it; third finger, close it; fourth finger, close it. Repeat this sequence; be sure to open each finger completely. Continue for 2 minutes.

PART FIVE

Time: 2 Minutes

Lie on the stomach. Place the hands under the shoulders, palms flat; lift the head, chest and chin, Cobra Pose. Stick the tongue all the way out, slowly breathe through the mouth, long and deep. Continue for 2 minutes.

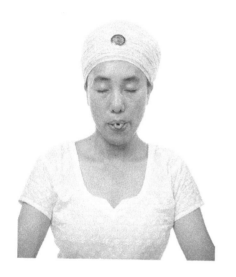

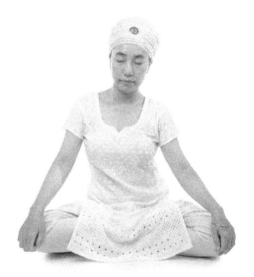

PART SIX

Time: 3.5 Minutes

Sit in Easy Pose with a straight spine. Curl the sides of the tongue up to make a U. Extend the tip of the tongue beyond the lips. Inhale through the rolled tongue and exhale through the nose, *Sitalee Praanayam*. Continue for 3.5 minutes.

PART SEVEN

52 Repetitions each direction

Sit in Easy Pose with the hands on the knees. Rotate the hips in a circular motion, grinding the pelvis, keep the spine lifted, and head level, Sufi Grind.

After 52 repetitions, switch directions. Continue for 52 repetitions.

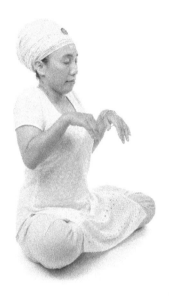

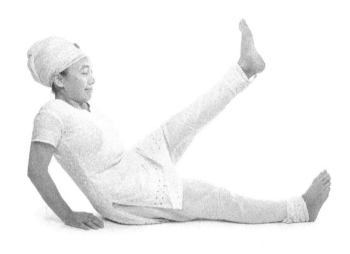

PART EIGHT

Time: 3 Minutes

Remain in Easy Pose. Bend the elbows, keep them relaxed at the sides. Bring the hands in front the body, relax the wrists and allow the hands to hang loosely. Roll the shoulders forward. Continue for 3 minutes.

PART NINE

Time: 3 Minutes

Remain seated, stretch the legs straight forward. Place the hands on ground just behind the hips. Raise alternate legs, bring the knee to the nose and back down; do not bend the knee. Continue for 3 minutes.

Comments: This affects the lower spine and if done properly will open up the sinuses.

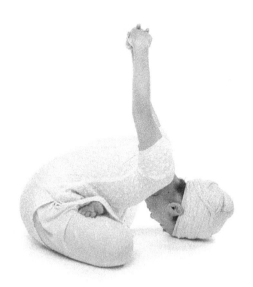

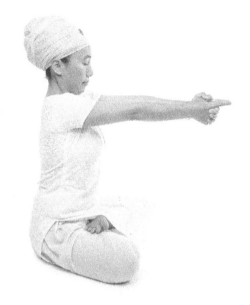

PART TEN

Time: 2 Minutes

Sit in Lotus Pose. Interlock the hands behind the back, lower the forehead forward to the ground. Raise the arms up. Be very peaceful.

After 2 minutes, chant HEALTHY AM I, HAPPY AM I, HOLY AM I. Continue for 1 minute.

To End: Inhale, stretch the arms up. Relax the arms down.

PART ELEVEN

Time: 3 Minutes

Remain in Lotus Pose. Stretch the arms forward, parallel to the ground. Interlace the fingers, extend the Jupiter Fingers (index fingers) together and straight pointing forward. Keep the spine and elbows straight. Breath is not specified. Continue for 3 minutes.

Comments: This kriya balances the aura and electromagnetic field, stimulates the elimination of toxins, develops muscular coordination, and gives balance to the brain. It is a great practice for staying in tune, particularly if you have something to do that requires quick, clear decisions. It is also excellent to practice if your work gives you brain fatigue and mental sluggishness. Exercises 1 through 4 balance the aura, muscles, and brain. Exercises 3 and 4 are especially good for brain balance. In fact, Exercise 3 was used as part of a system of therapy for the mentally imbalanced. Exercises 5 through 8 work on breaking up the deposits and releasing tension caused by poor digestion and high toxicity. Exercises 9 and 10 open the head and lung areas. Exercise 11 consolidates your mental projection into a one pointed positivity toward yourself and your daily tasks.

Meditation Flow of the Essence of Knowledge

June 20, 1994

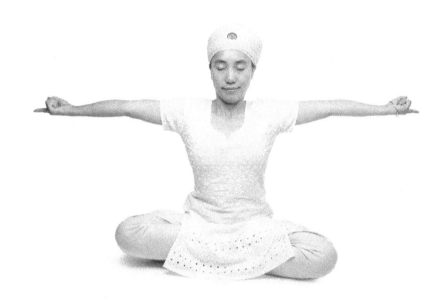

Sit in Easy Pose with a straight spine.

PART ONE

Time: 3 Minutes

Bring the arms straight out to the sides, parallel to the ground, Jupiter Fingers (index fingers) straight out, hold the rest of the fingers down with the thumbs, palms face forward, wrists straight. Stretch the chest out. Move the arms in small backward circles from the shoulders. Only the shoulder socket moves.

Move fast. Continue for 3 minutes.

To End: Inhale, hold the breath for 15 seconds and tighten the body, stretch the arms and Jupiter Fingers out, squeeze. Cannon Fire exhale. Repeat two more times. Relax.

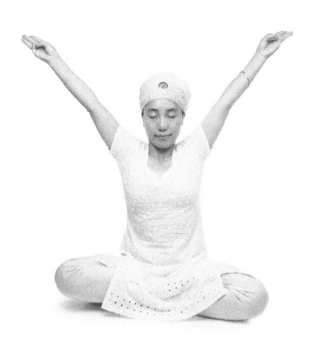

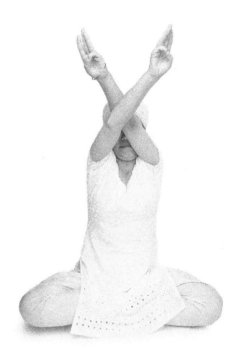

PART TWO

Time: 3 Minutes

Remain in Easy Pose. Hold the Mercury Fingers (pinky fingers) down with the thumbs, keep the rest of the fingers straight. Raise the arms up and move in a criss-cross motion in front of the face, alternate which arm crosses over the other. Move fast.

After 1 minute, add Breath of Fire to the movement. Continue for 2 minutes.

To End: Inhale deep, hold the breath for 5 seconds and move as fast as possible. Exhale. Inhale deep, hold the breath for 15 seconds and move the arms as fast as possible. Cannon Fire exhale. Repeat two more times. Relax.

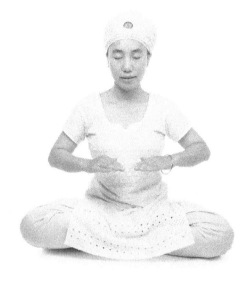

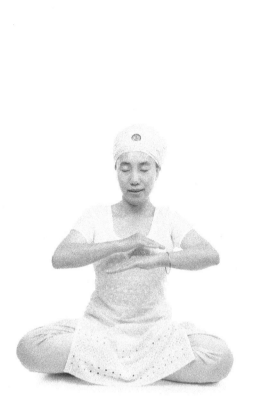

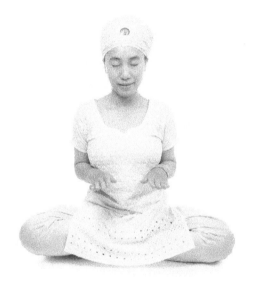

PART THREE

Time: 3.5 Minutes

Remain in Easy Pose. Bend the elbows, forearms forward, parallel to the ground, palms face each other. Move the hands in and out of fists, thumbs on the outside, quickly.

After 30 seconds, Cup the hands, fingers and thumbs together, move the hands around each other in small fast forward circles in front of the Heart Center. Chant HAR on every turn with the Tip of the Tongue as fast as possible. Loud. Continue for 3 minutes.

To End: Inhale, hold the breath for 20 seconds, hands stop moving. Turn the tip of the tongue up and back in the mouth, toward the throat, press the upper palate, hold tight. Cannon Fire exhale. Repeat two more times. Relax.

PART FOUR

Time: 1 Minute

Remain in Easy Pose. Bend the elbows, forearms parallel to the ground, hands relaxed, palms face down. Swing the elbows away from the body then with force in to hit the rib cage. Chant SAA and hit the rib cage, chant TAA as the elbows move out, chant NAA and hit the rib cage, chant MAA as the elbows move out. One complete cycle takes 2 seconds. Continue for 1 minute. Immediately begin Part Five.

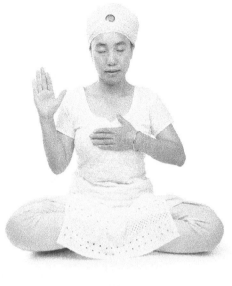

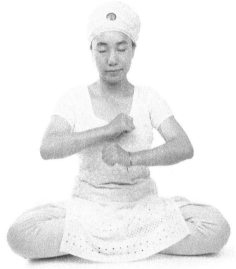

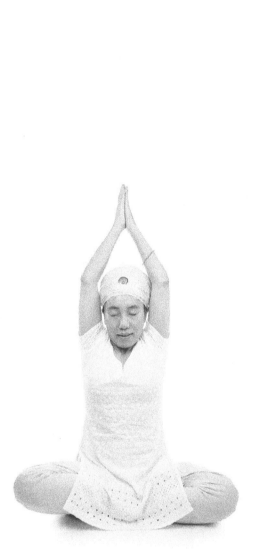

PART FIVE

Time: 4 Minutes

Remain in Easy Pose. Bring the hands together in Prayer Pose. Raise the arms up, elbows in toward the head; stretch up. Relax the breath. Play *Bole So Nihal*, "the oldest tape", keep stretching the hands up and sing with the music.

After 2 minutes, stand up, keep the arms extended overhead, palms together. Dance, jump. Continue for 2 minutes. Music ends. Immediately begin Part Six.

PART SIX

Time: 7 Minutes

Sit in Easy Pose with a straight spine. Place the left hand on the Heart Center, fingers together point right parallel to the ground, thumb relaxed. Bend the right elbow, relaxed by the side. Bring the right hand by the shoulder like taking an oath, fingers point up, palm faces forward. Close the eyes, look at the chin, Moon Center. The frontal lobe (forehead) will become heavy like lead. Consolidate and meditate. After 4.0 minutes meditate and sing with *Guru Dev Matta, Guru Dev Pitta*. Continue for 13 minutes.

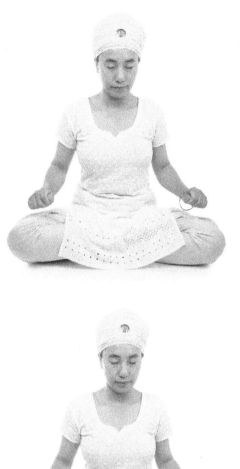

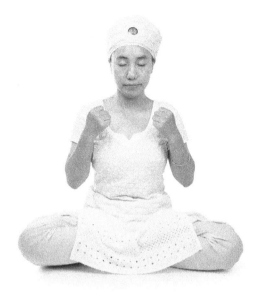

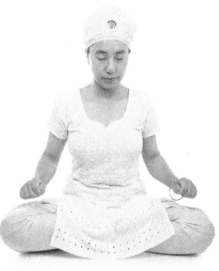

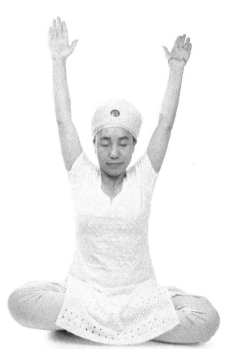

To End: Music ends. Inhale deep, hold for 5 seconds. Exhale. Inhale, hold the breath for 5 seconds and make fists, bend elbows 90 degrees, fists in front of the body, move the fists in small fast outward circles. Exhale. Relax the breath, hit the thighs with the palms for 5 seconds, hit the upper chest with fists for 5 seconds, cross the arms, hit opposite shoulders with flat hands for 5 seconds. Inhale, hold the breath for 5 seconds and stretch the arms straight up. Exhale, relax.

ARADHANA

An Experiential Journey

Years after our first experience of practicing *Sadhana*, whether from a written source or our teacher's actual voice, we begin to understand the significance, depth, and value of the teachings. With time, the constant practice and dedication and an exploratory spirit gradually build the neural connections for the comprehension to happen. During this time, the support of a teacher is advisable. Through the experience of this technology, the teacher can translate the teachings to the student so that the student can vibrate the frequency of the teachings and pass them to others.

In *Sadhana*, we start the journey to get to know ourselves. We establish the basis for the awakening to happen through discipline. In *Aradhana*, the journey continues revealing new horizons and new challenges. First, we look at the critical faculties and attitudes required for the transformation. Each topic includes an introduction to and instructions for a meditative kriya that supports understanding the theme. They make our journey within *Aradhana* an experiential one.

We have soul, we have divinity, and we have duality. In the Age of Aquarius, we can be our own teachers when we understand who we are. When we can see both divinity and duality simultaneously, then we know ourselves. We accept all of whom we are and are liberated while yet alive. Without authority, there is no self-realization.

Kriya to Balance the Glandular System

April 2, 1996

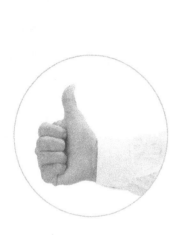

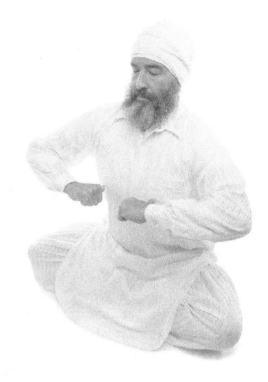

PART ONE

Sit in Easy Pose with a straight spine.

Mudra: Bend the Jupiter (index), Saturn (middle), Sun (ring) and Mercury (pinky) fingers in to touch the center of the palm. Apply a firm pressure; it will be painful. Thumbs are relaxed. Raise the arms to the level of the Heart Center; bend the elbows to bring the hands toward each other in front of the chest, forearms parallel to the ground, palms face down. Keep the chest open and the arms strong and tense, especially the bicep muscles. This mudra is not recommended if you have arthritis in your hands.

Breath: Inhale and exhale through the nose. Inhale and exhale through the mouth. Continue this breath cycle alternating nasal breath and mouth breath.

Eye Focus: There is no specified eye focus.

Time: Continue for 11 minutes. Immediately begin Part 2.

Comments: Use the muscles in your arms, hands and fingers. The muscles may become tired, but if you continue you will gain strength. After two minutes, you will feel changes internally as the pituitary secretions direct changes in the muscular and glandular systems.

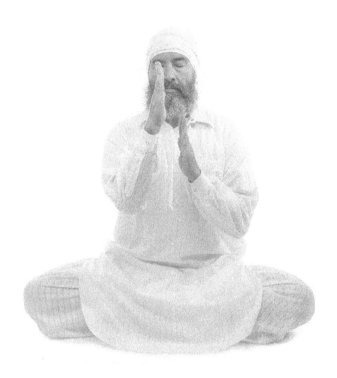

Remain in Easy Pose.

Mudra: Raise the right hand in front of the face with the thumb tip at the level of the Tip of the Nose, palm facing left. Raise the left hand, palm facing right, so that the fingertips are at the level of the base of the right palm. Hands are separately slightly. Fingers are straight and relaxed.

Breath: Breathe consciously, long and deep for the first 8 minutes.

Eye Focus: Close the eyes.

Mantra: After 8 minutes, begin to chant *Humee Hum Brahm Hum* (version by Nirinjan Kaur is played) for 3 minutes.

Time: Continue for 8 minutes then 3 Minutes chanting for a total of 11 minutes.

To End: Inhale, hold the breath and shake your head as powerfully you can, shake it like a mad person for 15 seconds. Exhale and relax. If you are with others, talk with each other in order to bring yourself back.

Comments: Maintain a balance with the hands and allow yourself to dissolve as a bubble dissolves within the ocean. You regenerate yourself as you merge with the One.

Calm After the Storm

Life is like a stormy ocean. By following a spiritual path on this journey, some acquire the flexibility and sensitivity to allow change. Every change is like a small death; it is necessary to make room for rebirth. Only through a continuous renewal can this life journey be lived at its fullest.

What drives human beings to transform their own lives and seek their essence? We feel that we can no longer proceed as we are. We feel that something is missing, and we are suffering, feeling separated, longing to belong to a higher way of existence. Whatever the reason, the real or imaginary motivation strengthens our resolve to change our lives. The process of change starts when we understand that we are both the creative source and the vibratory nucleus of the space in which we live. Our environment, the quality of our life and relationships, all originate, as we have seen, from our vibratory frequency, and change is the work of our inner Self, projected outwards.

Every stage of life has its blessings, as well as challenges. The cycles of growth continuously present us with new opportunities. External influences lead us to inevitable change. Why not, then, consciously prepare for change, welcome, and not fight it? Daily practice facilitates internal change as we become more aware. It is the transition from being a yoga philosopher to being a yogi. The information learned leads us to change. Through *Sadhana*, we discipline ourselves so that our body and mind can serve our soul to express the Infinite in any situation.

Through discipline, we consciously create the time and space to observe our subconscious mind's beliefs and reactionary patterns. We deliberately put ourselves in the observer role, witnessing the reactive and compulsive instincts, which resist change. Paradoxically, reactivity, often mistaken for sensitivity, makes us progressively less attentive to possible transformation, while discipline keeps us connected to reality. Through practice, we begin to see the motivations of our actions and build our creative potential. Thanks to the daily cleaning of the unconscious mind, the conscious mind prevails and handles the flow of thoughts with more authority. We are able to recognize the effects of identification with a thought and to let go of one thought and choose a more elevated one. No longer influenced by the past, we are conscious of the present and consciously affecting the future.

The cleaning of the subconscious represents a key passage in our growth process. Temporary metabolic obstructions (blocks of the subconscious that prevent clear communication between the conscious and super-conscious mind) do not disappear. They gradually surface as the incoherence between the subconscious world and the conscious one, between the internal intention and the external projection. This is a delicate period when the subconscious still resists consistent daily practice.

With the subconscious finally empty, a new and unconditional horizon opens for us. Discipline prevails, the subconscious accepts our practice of *Sadhana*, and the body follows. With our *Sadhana* established, we reach *Aradhana*. After a long climb, arriving at a mountain lake grants calmness and relief, so in *Aradhana*, we find ourselves in a cozy, peaceful space. The time and sleep we sacrificed turns out to be our most profitable investment. Everything is in a state of balance where we appreciate and live gratefully every moment of the day. In *Aradhana*, discipline is satisfying. Uncomfortable sensations or resistance that surface come from our willingness to keep growing and changing. It is still possible to be bewitched by the old frequencies, strong enough to lead to an impasse. Only a tiny step divides us from the peak of consciousness to returning to our old identification and need for emotional satisfaction. Our practice can become either an experience that elevates, joyful and new every time, or a source of frustration and tiredness.

Thus, it is not opening a door and then closing it, thinking the job is done. Without continuous renewed commitment, the strongest of practices becomes a sterile mechanical action, and we inevitably return to the old idea of ourselves, as well as our emotional desires. For this reason, in *Aradhana*, we must remember our path and never lose sight of our destination. We risk thinking during the journey that the acquired habit of waking up and doing the practice is our primary intention. We may be reluctant to awaken new and deeper experiences through silent contemplation. There is nothing sadder than filling our time in a dull, ritualistic way. Many of us have experienced this fragile point, sometimes using it to justify giving up the process. The world that awaits us is unknown, requiring powerful motivation to keep us moving forward. Only perseverance aligned with rediscovering and recommitting to our primary intentions can lead us to our source of strength and inspiration.

In *Aradhana's* crisis, we feel we are halfway from what we thought we were and what we really are. We are neither happy nor unhappy, neither spiritual nor earthly. From this uncertainty, we may believe that our previous situation was better. We do not understand that if we fall now, we fall without our old personality as a safety net. Thus, we have three choices: either we can keep on suffering in a state of doubt, we can anesthetize ourselves by going back, or we can decide to go ahead into the unknown. With the first two options, we become stagnant. Stagnation is a contraction that solidifies the entranced state from the Age of Pisces. In this hypnotic state, we dream of waking up from the dream. We are unable to identify who we really are and act from this alternative version of ourselves. With the third option, we leave insecurities and false identification behind to live freely. We find mastery.

Even after we have gotten to know ourselves and live a conscious life, the mind talks to us unrestrained, and the subconscious tempts us. Crisis arrives unexpectedly. All the hard work done to relate and entrust the Infinite seems to vanish, eclipsed by a situation, which is emotional and neurotic. Life and growth ask us to find our motivation and decide to commit again. The subconscious lures us with the illusion of encountering something special that we never experienced before and promising emotional satisfaction. While all this happens, it is not easy to recall the complete satisfaction gained from our commitments rather the transitory pleasure coming from the illusion.

Yogic technology teaches us that there are three aspects to cultivate to face these challenges. First: the discipline to develop our consciousness through devotion and the sacrifice of routine dynamics. Second: the tenacity of not giving up or feeling defeated, rather considering lost battles as experience and a means to victory. Third: abandoning self-criticism, a sense of inadequacy, guilt, or shame, in order to discover the potential hidden in any circumstance. It is not important to become perfect, but rather to set a goal, which is greater than we are now. In the turbulence of the crisis and under the pressure of the challenge, it is of utmost importance to look deeper to find again the motivation that led us to where we are now and draw from it the strength to go on.

Each one of us has had their reason to start and gradually commit to Sadhana. Feeling hopeless, and feeling the urge to identify oneself in the spirit, is maybe the strongest motivation to encourage you on the yogic path. It is fundamental to the yoga practice to feel compassion for ourselves, which can only be achieved by re-balancing ourselves daily. Compassion is a vital tool to overcome the crisis of conscious, mental and spiritual growth. Compassion is the mother of courage and the first step to forget and forgive. If we do not let go, it means we are unable to forget and forgive, and we lose grace and integrity. We maintain grace through discipline, and integrity by our *Sadhana*. To reach the goal of yoga, to live a conscious life (one devoted to honoring the altitude and mission of our superior Self, not influenced by the opposites, living our originality to serve) can become complex and feel impossible. We must not compromise what we have or could have.

In *Aradhana*, the inability to evoke and keep mental silence, to stay in the *Shuniya*, is the alarm bell, which warns us about an imminent or already existing crisis. Recognizing it depends on how alert we are to perceive silence, despite a constant flow of thoughts. After years of practice, *Shuniya* should be accessible in every moment of our life, not only when we sit to meditate or practice. The inability to do this reminds us that our practice's quality has decreased, while we remember that this regression is also a natural part of the journey. The *condicio sine qua non* is mental silence: *Shuniya*. Only from here can we build a relationship with our practice, ourselves, and our environment.

Often this reveals an uncertainty with the teachings and the Golden Chain. Without this connection, sailing through the spaces of consciousness is uncertain.

Kriya to Create Strength of Character

October 9, 1990

There are many spiritual paths, *dharmas* or religions and many saints, sages and gurus. To be successful on any path with any guide requires that you have spirit. Spirit comes from the strength of discipline and discipline is vital to grasp reality.

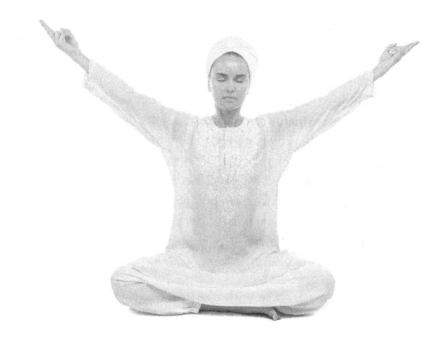

PART ONE

Sit in Easy Pose with a straight spine.

Mudra: Extend the Jupiter (index) and Saturn (middle) fingers straight and hold the Sun (ring) and Mercury (pinky) fingers down with the thumbs. Raise the arms out to the sides and up to 30 degrees angle from the shoulder line, elbows are straight, palms face up. Pressure will be on the elbows.

Breath: Unspecified.

Eye Focus: Close the eyes.

Mantra:
ARDAAS BHAEE AMAR DAAS GUROO AMAR DAAS GUROO ARDAS BHAEE

RAAM DAAS GUROO RAAM DAAS GUROO RAAM DAAS GUROO SACHEE SAHEE

Listen and whistle to the instrumental version of this mantra.

Time: Continue for 11 minutes.

To End: Music ends. Inhale deeply, raise the arms overhead, lock the hands, and pull yourself up, stretch up, elbows are straight. Exhale and relax. Immediately begin Part 2.

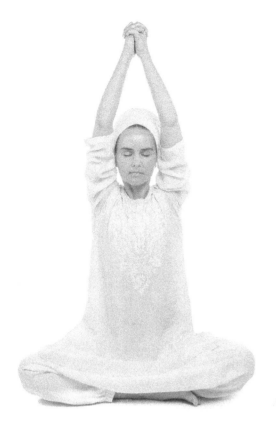

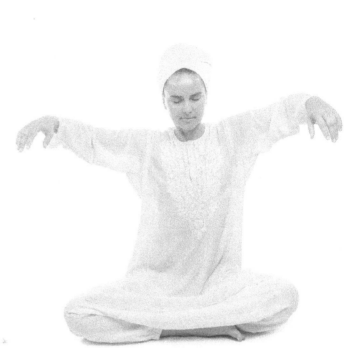

PART TWO

Remain in Easy Pose.

Mudra: Come into the same posture as in Part 1.

Breath: Breathe Long and Deep.

Eye Focus: Eyes remain closed.

Mantra: Same as Part 1.

Time: After 7 minutes, maintain the posture and listen to the instrumental version of the mantra. Continue for 4 minutes.

To End: Music stops. Inhale deeply, hold the breath and stretch up for 15 seconds while feeling every positive feeling – successful, competent, blissful, whatever comes to you; let these qualities be ingrained in you. Exhale and relax.

PART THREE

Remain in Easy Pose.

Mudra: Move the shoulders, arms and body wildly with the music.

Breath: Unspecified.

Music: *Punjabi Drums*

Eye Focus: Unspecified.

Time: Continue for 5 minutes.

To End: Music stops. Inhale deeply; put the hands on the Heart Center one over the other. Close the eyes and relax the breath. Maintain the posture. Immediately begin Part 4.

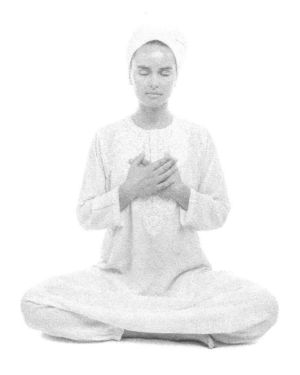

PART FOUR

Remain in Easy Pose.

Mudra: Maintain the hands on the Heart Center.

Breath: Breathe long and deep. Meditate.

Eye Focus: Eyes remain closed.

Mantra: Mul Mantra

EK ONG KAAR, SAT NAAM, KARTAA PURKH, NIRBHO, NIRVAIR, AKAAL MOORAT, AJOONEE, SAIBUNG, GUR PRASAAD, JAAP, AAD SUCH, JUGAAD SUCH, HAIBHEE SUCH, NANAK HOSEE BHEE SUCH

Time: Continue for 5 minutes (in the original class the gong was played ending with 3 distinct strong strikes just below center). Then meditate for 1 minute in silence. Continue meditating for 3 minutes, listening to the Mul Mantra (a classic Indian version was played in class). The music stops. Inhale deeply. Exhale. Resume the music and chant, copying the sound. Continue for 3 minutes.

Being in the State of Non-Existence

In *Aradhana*, we continuously experience an infinite horizon. The daily practice creates a state of consciousness in which time and space constraints do not affect. Mental calmness leaves room for a total vacuum; nothing influences us. We exist and non-exist at the same time, and non-existence is the practical experience of the Infinite.

Through *Sadhana*, we achieve union through a gradual and slow journey. This marriage happens in silence and through silence, with a consciousness that nullifies the ego. It is possible to experience being without polarization. The mind selects and rejects polarities. We get to zero, in alignment with the One, which is our support. This dynamic is a description and, at the same time, the goal of yoga. Asana, mantra, mudra, and pranayama are all part of yogic technology to guide us to experience *Shuniya*.

From this universality of purpose, it is interesting to look at our school's approach, which recognizes in Patanjali a guide for a reality that would exist two thousand years after it was written. Patanjali described the meditative process and the resulting state in a concise and clear way, almost scientifically: "When the mind, applied to meditation, becomes unintentional, the presumption to act stops."[1] The mind eliminates other objects or thoughts from its attention to devote itself to a single object and gradually illuminates it by penetrating its fundamental nature: this is cognitive enstasis (enstasis: union, totality, absorption in something, total concentration of the spirit, conjunction). With this complete spiritual focus, all other mental functions cease. In time the introverted and extroverted mental functions dissolve, and we reach the non-cognitive enstasis. With an empty mind, the only thing left is the subject, purified from its object: pure spirit, the motionless seer that continues to inhabit the empty mind.

In the second four limbs of yoga – *Pratyahara, Dharana, Dhyana*, and *Samadhi* – Patanjali describes the essence of yoga and its goal. He highlights the need to use motionlessness to inhibit the mental functions to solve the duality of attraction/aversion related to thoughts without its outward mental functions. Only in silence can we understand reality. The process to reach the state of Shuniya is not a cognitive, intellectual, or rational process, and it does not come through study or mere knowledge. It comes from the constant observation and exploration of one's own mind, getting to know it so deeply that we take it to a neutral level. To know by receiving undistorted input and sensations. "Know your mind, and you'll know the whole universe", said Guru Nanak. Because of this, Rishis, Yogis, and Spiritual Masters were able to explain the experience of reality without modern scientific understanding.

By meditating during the ambrosial hours, we conquer the universe effortlessly. Effort is required in sacrificing the "I think therefore I am", in favor of "I don't think therefore I am not". It is only through non-existence, from which everything originates, that we can relate, hear and understand. Being in the state of non-existence, we balance our lives. Non-existence is necessary to benefit from merging in the Infinite.

How do we enter into and live in the state of *Shuniya*? The first answer from Kundalini Yoga's technology is to apply the negative mind and deny the thought and stop its progress. Then use discrimination to transcend it. Another way is to apply the positive mind and utilize sound waves to deter thoughts and cut them so that the sound prevails over the train of thoughts. The negative mind uses the Shakti force, and the positive mind uses a devotional Bhakti attitude.

A third approach is the pure contemplation of the contents of the experience at a precise moment. Nothing is denied, nothing is proposed, and all is contained within the observer's contemplative space. Being steady in a non-acting way dissolves any block resulting in the experience of silence. The neutral mind

[1] Patanjali, Yoga sutras

expands and moves in a Shakti and Bhakti equilibrium. To reach *Shuniya*, we need to absorb the concept of "I am, I am not" and accept this coexistence of being and not being. We need to experience "non-being" to balance "being".

The clear sensation of stillness we have during practice is not something to produce but to experience. *Shuniya*, emptiness, is always present beneath the flow of thoughts, the recklessness, the anxiety, the confusion, and stress; we just need to allow ourselves to listen and be with it. The state of silence is not always the same; the quality and intensity depending on how much you are willing to listen. Silence has no limitations; only the practitioners can limit themselves. In *Shuniya*, non-existence "I am not" prevails over "I am". On the contrary, however, when we believe the subconscious, the subconscious controls us through dreams, memories, anticipations, and assumptions. In this context, it is interesting to explore this kind of a *'hypnotic state'*, in which you experience everything but reality. To acknowledge and break this state, it is necessary to go to the source of the problem: humans find it hard to accept their higher Self. When we do not accept it, even though it is real, we take a false alternative. This is our way of "saving face".

We see this in social life where people are recognized by their "status" based on profession, wealth, social background instead of being recognized as human beings. When we deny our true Self, then life is devoid of vastness, breadth, vision, courage, and there will be no other way left to go but to qualify ourselves. Then our life justifies our limited self, rather than being the higher Self. The lack of relationship with our essence is evident from our education, lifestyle, and our priorities. We have been educated to live with the anxiety of accumulating and with the intent to achieve a certain status. In this hypnotic state, we live in a bubble of restricted consciousness, with no vision of reality, in which we become enslaved, senseless, and robotic. We find ourselves at a dead-end, repetitively experiencing one of life's polarities. It is like consuming energy without refueling, exhaling without inhaling. We strive to own and to do; we are existing, not living. We become neurotic. We listen superficially, relate inadequately and perceive and act ignorantly. The suffering this causes becomes unbearable. The change into the Age of Aquarius with its pressure of so much information contributes heavily to *self-hypnosis*. We dream of waking up from a dream, a dream in a dream, a double fantasy in which we believe our hypnosis is the means to reality. What lies beneath the hypnosis is an intact human being, the authentic Self, divine and radiant like God.

We are not wrong nor imperfect. We do not have to become something different. Nothing comes from outside; everything is already within us. We are just not able to accept who we are. By practicing *Sadhana*, we acknowledge and dissolve the hypnosis and enter *Aradhana*. We begin to explore life as a free person, having discovered the power of non-action. In *Sadhana*, we consciously try to be in every gesture, breath, and sound, not to escape from something but to become influenced by it. We do not wait for time to pass. Instead, we create a momentum within the moment.

Two blocks nurture resistance to surrendering in *Shuniya* and leave the spell intact – the non-willingness to forgive and to forget – and we betray ourselves. Let us forget the memories, the uncomfortable contents of the subconscious, and our preconceptions. There is no way to experience the reality without forgiving and forgetting. In Western culture, surrender and compliance are weaknesses, while in the spiritual world, they are seen as two extraordinary forces. The seed needs to surrender to the soil to become a tree.

Kriya Existence from Non-Existence (Pratyahara, I am Not)

November 1, 1994

Almost everyone lives in the state of self-hypnosis, unconscious and unbalanced, wanting without unwanting, insecure without security. This kriya helps to find the polarity.

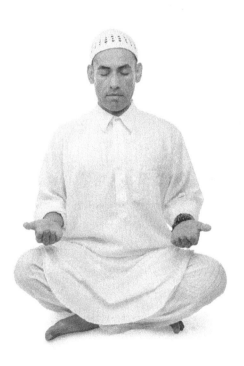
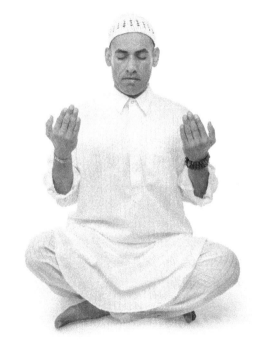

PART ONE A

Sit in Easy Pose with a straight spine.

Mudra: Bend the elbows with the arms pointing forward; forearms are parallel to the ground. Cup the hands, thumbs relaxed and palms facing up. Keep the upper arms locked against the body. Move both hands up and down; the motion is precise and sharp from the elbow. Isolate the movement like an electric shock creating an upward jerking motion of the forearms and hands.

Breath: Breathe naturally.

Eye focus: Focus the eyes at the Tip of the Nose

Time: Continue for 5 minutes. Keep the moving the arms and begin Part 1B.

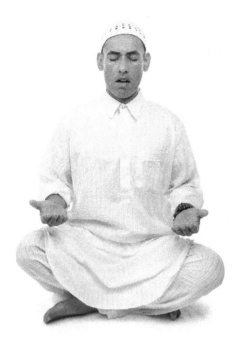

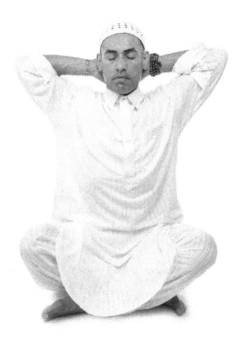

PART ONE B

Remain in Easy Pose.

Mudra: Maintain the posture and continue the movement with added breath focus.

Breath: As the hands come up, exhale through the mouth as if blowing out a candle, quickly and powerfully. The inhale will automatically happen. Breathe simultaneously with the movement.

Eye Focus: Maintain the focus on the Tip of the Nose.

Time: Continue for 5 minutes.

To End: Inhale deeply, suspend the breath for 12 seconds, become thoughtless. Exhale; suspend the breath out for 12 seconds, breathing out all thoughts. I am not. Inhale and immediately begin Part 2.

Comment: On each exhale push out all disease, all negative habits. Stay alert; resist the tendency to give up.

PART TWO

Remain in Easy Pose.

Mudra: Maintain the posture with the upper arms pressed against the body, elbows bent and forearms parallel to the ground. The hands cupped and the palms face up. There is no movement.

Breath: Unspecified.

Eye Focus: Unspecified.

Mental Focus: Meditate on zero, I am not, be in the state of Shuniya.

Time: Continue for 15 minutes.

To End: Inhale deeply, lock your hands behind your neck and powerfully twist toward the right as far as possible. Hold tight for 20 seconds. Return to center and exhale. Inhale deeply again and twist to the left as far as possible. Hold tight for 20 seconds. Return to center and exhale. Inhale deep, move the head backward as

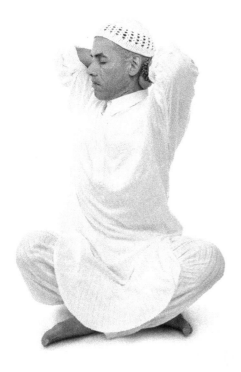

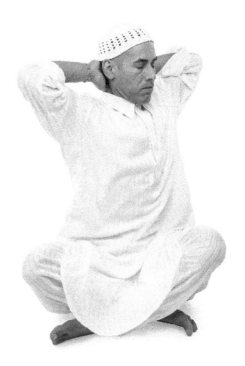

much as possible, hold for 20 seconds. Return to center, exhale and relax.

Comments: Prosperity depends on balance; something always comes from nothing. Life leads to death and death to new life; this is the natural cycle. Enjoy the freedom of not being. Repeat to yourself: "I am not, I am not the body, not the mind, not the soul, not the existence".

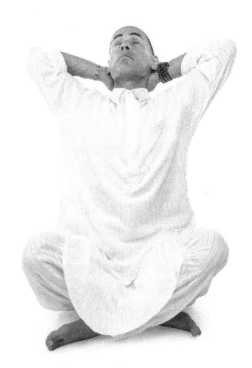

THE CONNECTION WITH THE GOLDEN CHAIN THROUGH THE SUBTLE BODY

The teachings of Kundalini Yoga consist of the combined consciousness of the Masters who have come before us. Collectively, we refer to this lineage as the "Golden Chain". Guru Ram Das granted all practitioners of Kundalini Yoga the connection with that flow of consciousness. The acknowledgment of Guru Ram Das as the main link in the Golden Chain comes through Baba Siri Chand, Guru Nanak's son, a Baal Yogi, who kept his sixteen-year-old appearance even when he was a hundred and sixty. He was head of an important ascetic yoga school, when he bowed to Guru Ram Das acknowledging him as the holder of the throne of Raj Yoga. The Sikh consciousness enriched Kundalini Yoga. This ancient practice no longer was exclusive to kings or ascetics but recognized the royalty and sovereignty in every human, taught and practiced by all, even those living an active family life, working, and part of their community. [2]

We set aside differentiation, rationality, and egotism with the protection of this consciousness flow, like taking off our shoes before entering a temple. With devotion in our hearts, we bring our intention as an offering in front of

[2] The Heart of the Teacher, lecture by Guru Dev Singh and Gurucharan Singh, Assisi, Italy 2004

the altar, as if bowing our head to a Master. Our relationship with the Golden Chain is one of lineage and legacy. Lineage denotes those who were together temporally before us or will be in the future due to tradition or initiation. They can be family members or belong to the same spiritual school. Legacy is what we have by birthright, not due to blood ties, but to destiny. Through the ages, the vital factor in transmitting these teachings has been an elevated state of consciousness. Every link in the chain increased the consciousness to the level required for the teachings to continue to spread, whether through the son of a King, a Guru, an orphan, or an untouchable. Any person who would want to be part of the lineage must increase his or her consciousness to the legacy level. The Golden Chain honors the lineage and serves the legacy. Lineage and legacy are two polarities coexisting in a creative tension. There is no solution. The question is how much we are willing to flow with it, accept its privileges and duties, and create the conditions to enter into the stream of the Golden Chain and become the teachings themselves. Kundalini Yoga technology gives us a chance to call upon this legacy through the quality and vastness of our consciousness. We access this immense heritage through our devotion and commitment to *Sadhana*, the study and practice of the technology, and the attitude to serve the mission. Lineage is not required; everyone who has practiced even just one Kundalini Yoga class has the opportunity to connect to the Golden Chain.

This is not a ritualistic connection. It comes from the willingness to merge with the flow of consciousness and to experience the transformative energy. This connection allows us to practice and teach authentically, dropping the personality and ego to share the power of the Golden Chain. The entry code is the Adi Mantra: *Ong Namo Guru Dev Namo*. It is the first technology for students and teachers to direct their minds and immerse themselves in the Golden Chain. Its attentive and precise vocalization, supported by an intention and a projection, directly stimulates the kundalini to rise. Merging with the Adi Mantra makes us receptive and sensitive. We enter shuniya. The subtle body travels to the ethers and accesses the wisdom from the teachers who came before us. The five etheric levels are different states of energetic realms. While still alive, we can connect and relate the ethers through our etheric capacity.[3]

How does the consciousness move in the Adi Mantra? Chanting Ong evokes a suspension of our intellectual activity and mental functions to promote the state of *Shuniya*. The sound *Ong* echoes like the vibration of a gong. As the root of the tongue touches the back of the throat, the reverberation of the "*ng*" is experienced in the nasal cavity and the frontal lobe. The recitation of Ong creates connection without attachment providing for essential neutrality for creating

[3] The Aquarian Teacher, Life Cycles and Life Style Textbook, pp 44, published by Kundalini Research Institute, 2010.

The Five Blue Ethers

Once the soul and the subtle body trespass the earth's electromagnetic field, they're ready to go through the five blue ethers.

The first blue ether, *Karta Purakh*, contains the Akashic Register where there's all the information on the universe and the life stories of all beings. When we go through this first state, our individual story is poured into this "cosmic file", and through reincarnation our subtle body receives the imprinting given by our previous karmas.

In the second blue ether, *Sopurak*, we evaluate what is our position and which lessons we still have to learn in order to make our consciousness go forward. We are given a test on these lessons and we need to show we can do it by staying constant and neutral through the different challenges our soul has to go through.

The passage between one and the other of these reigns doesn't automatically happen, it requires us to complete and internal process, as well as reaching the purification level, always higher than our consciousness. We are not alone then, but according to our spiritual orientation, there's a guide to light our path.

The third blue ether, *Purakh*, is an etheric reign. We get there after facing our karma and receiving the tools to cancel it. Once we overcome the lessons of space and time, we move in a much elevated space which leads us to an individual identity of the infinite Self. What drives our consciousness once we get to this state, it's service and blessing. There are no barriers between the third and fourth stadium.

The fourth blue ether, *Brahm Prakash*, is the kingdom of Radiance, where we experiment bliss. In the fourth blue ether we enter the universal flow of consciousness which connects all living beings. In this state the subtle body is still present, but it won't in the firth one, where we'll experience a total fusion with the Infinite Self.

The fifth blue ether, *Brahm* or God, is the total union with God. In this kingdom we are beyond the limits of existence forms, in a space of absolute bliss, where we experiment the divine gaze of the Creator. The soul of Guru Ram Das, as the of our Master, is united in the infinite Self in the fifth ether, but through the subtle body, which resides in the fourth ether, they can guide us and be our constant source of spiritual richness.

an effective and genuine relationship. The vibratory approach offers the link to experience the flow from the Infinite to the finite teacher. Chanting *Namo*, we throw the seed of intention to create and hold the space for the Golden Chain. *Bija*, the seed, if planted in the state of *Shuniya*, is in total potentiality. We are in fourth ether with Namo, in the flow of the teachings; we enter it thanks to the honest intention of being teachers and students. *Namo* descends from the fourth ether to the third. The intention, facing the Master and the teachings, has the chance to be clear and concrete. At this moment, the mind serves and translates what the heart wants. The omni-directional nature of this intention is the real act of love toward the universe. *Namo* is like bowing. It is an attitude of respect and receptiveness, showing our dignity by acknowledging a higher consciousness.

With our willingness to be connected, *Guru Dev* reveals a contemplative listening space. We perceive the concentric waves of sound spreading, and we listen to the vibration of the seed while it grows and spreads. The attentive listening of the vibrated and vibrating sound wave increases the intention of connection. In the mastery of *Shuniya* within our destiny, we become a catalyst for people and possibilities. This is the phase of attention, which precedes that of the expansion.

We acquire a total vision, and we find the voice of God in everything we hear. We descend into the second ether with *Guru*. *Guru* is that which leads us from ignorance to wisdom, and *Dev* is the navigator. The connection is now solid. By vibrating the final *Namo*, we project the intention to expand. Everything is complete. Now the wisdom of the radiant body and the subtle body guides us in a personally impersonal way. The projection now has the impulse on a clear path.

Suspension – *Ong*, penetration – *Namo*, attention – *Guru Dev* and projection – *Namo* compose the path of the Adi Mantra. We are within the uninterrupted flow of the teachings and experience the tantric energy in this blessing.

Kriya Clarify the Subtle Body

October 11, 1996

The power of the Subtle Body is its ability to attract opportunities. When faced with the worst circumstances you act with grace and elevate yourself and Nature will serve you.

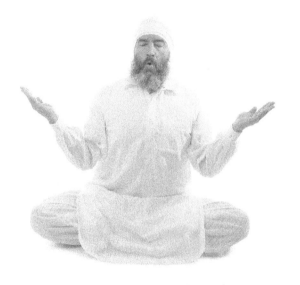

INSTRUCTIONS:

Sit in Easy Pose with a straight spine.

Mudra: Elbows are relaxed at the sides with the forearms parallel to the ground and out to the sides at a 45-degree angle. Palms face up, fingers together and relaxed. While you inhale through an "O" mouth, raise the hands over the top of the head, left fingers overlap and touch the right fingers, palms face downward. Create an arc over the head. Exhale through an "O" mouth and lower the hands to the original position. Move to the rhythm of Tantric Har, 1 movement up or down per second, a complete cycle takes 2 seconds. Pull the navel and diaphragm in with the exhalation.

Breath: Inhale and exhale through "O" mouth with movement of the hands.

Eye Focus: Unspecified.

Mantra: *Tantric HAR* is played to set the rhythm of the movement.

Time: Continue for 11 minutes.

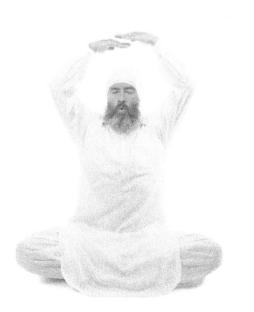

To End: Music stops. Inhale, suspend the breath, interlock the fingers and stretch the arms straight up, squeeze and stretch every muscle of the body, stretch for 15 seconds. Exhale and repeat 2 more times. Relax.

Comments: When you are comfortable practicing for 11 minutes, increase to 22 minutes and then to 31 minutes. Do not practice for more than 31 minutes.

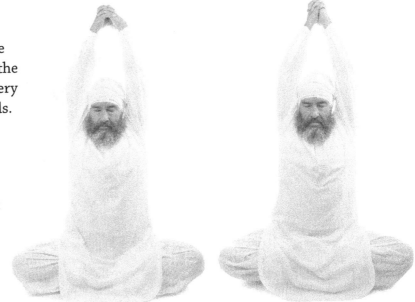

A Matter of Relation

In *Aradhana*, the time comes to practice what we have acquired in the internal process and express it into actions. We need to crystallize our psyche to express the experience into thoughts, words, and actions. From a philosophical level to the concreteness of living, the step from theory to practice consciously, naturally, completely changes the depth of our relationship with ourselves, with others, and with the environment. Throughout history, humans have challenged their limits to find themselves. The common idea has been that knowing ourselves is the path to happiness and success. This indomitable search for inner values and potential power has manifested differently in Eastern and Western cultures. In the East, they explored the internal realms of the mind and consciousness, while in the West, they explored places, lands unknown to them. Today the Western approach, including the exploration of new lands, is no longer possible. The entire world has been mapped, and every person is traceable by satellite. Modern Western explorers wanting to challenge themselves have no other choice but to go deep into the least known areas and lose themselves willingly or scientifically, regardless of the danger. For example, mountain climbers first climbed the highest peaks using oxygen, then later without oxygen. Next, they pushed themselves to climb mountains in quick succession, one after the other. Not enough of a challenge, the biggest competition then becomes not to climb but run, so the winner is the fastest person. The only possibility of real discovery lies in space or deep in the oceans.

Without taking away the fascination of exploration, today's real adventure is exploring one's own unknown, and from there, changing relationships. We live the adventure of a life externally focused, brave, and conscious only when we live our internal dimension with the same intensity. The internal life nurtures the external one. It is a mirror of it. Our outer drive is cultivated in the intimacy of consciousness. Every success comes from our capacity to relate with ourselves, others, and the universe. We have seen that Kundalini Yoga unifies the individual consciousness with the universal one, the individual human magnetic field and the universal one. Essentially, yoga is a connection that covers the distance caused by separation and unknowing.

The fundamental assumption in this process is dependent on the primary relation: the one with ourselves. If I cannot relate to my own Self, I cannot connect with others, so I cannot relate to the universe. Every suffering comes from the incapacity to have authentic and concrete relations. The yogi can relate to the Self, others, and everything. Comprehension and knowledge come from the experience that follows the intention to connect. Happiness arises from feeling one and at the same time unified, from not denying oneself or our surroundings, and feeling everything—the experience of being completely immersed in the reality of the relationship. What happens at that exact moment is impossible to say. It is extraordinary and requires a high level of containment and acceptance. In *Aradhana*, we consolidate our capacity, sensitivity, and intention to make this real. Through the sensory system of the Self, we connect the soul with the experience, reaching an understanding of this life.

When we first practice Kundalini Yoga, we use kriyas to relate to situations, others and our self. Each kriya has the technology of Kundalini Yoga condensed in it. Within the kriya, the sensations that arise are not influenced by our mind's judgments and belief systems. On the contrary, we interpret them in the reality of that moment. Thus, the mind, free from conditioning and preconceptions, can process and respond most appropriately based on the situation's reality. By observing the mind's judgment of what is right or wrong and accepting these polarities as diversities, we maintain neutrality. From this new perspective, we can see new opportunities wherever they exist. To live unconsciously is living a life of suffering; this is not your life. On the contrary, from the depth of the relations with ourselves and the universe, a mission surfaces from a vision, a glimpse of the unknown. The link to a life without insecurities and uncertainties comes with trust, courage, and intuition: invest in yourself by trusting the Infinite.

Everything in life exists as a relation: between you and your eyes reading these lines, between the unconscious process and the conscious one, between associations and differentiations. Subconscious tendencies impede the neutral experience. Kriya affects the subconscious to eliminate these obstructions. The success of a kriya depends on all aspects – the breath, mudra and mantra, concentration, immobility and movement, and how the body, through the senses, perceives the experience. The act of relating is the act of knowing and being known, to listening and being heard. The profound reality of being is known through relating to it.

The process of relating is an act of love, both terrifying and astounding at the same time. When the love for our Self allows self-forgiveness, accepting both our worst and best, it is possible to relate to someone else based on acceptance, rather than reaction or defense. We measure consciousness in progressive levels of love starting from emotional assumptions, and compensation needs to pure and unconditional love, which sees God and his will in everything. Love is a state of consciousness in which there are no obstacles to the interconnection, and in which we neither resist complete happiness nor suffering. When this happens, we realize that the experience of love is more extraordinary than its object; this is the transcending experience. Such a deep love can be extended to everything, because it does not depend on the person, but on the quality of the love given.

Kriya The Internal Force to Purify Actions

October 11, 1996

As humans, after we accomplish something, we tend to want to rest. It is not time to rest. It is not an end. It is rather a sign that we are just beginning. Every success is a new beginning, every day is a new day, and every moment is full of potential. The *totality of consciousness* comes when we fulfill our commitment and responsibility. When we know our true Identity, our actions become pure, and we recognize our purpose, our destiny – that is the goal of Kundalini Yoga.

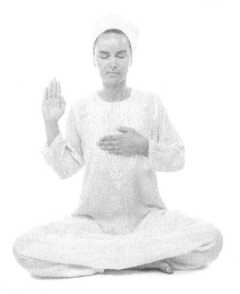

PART ONE

Sit in Easy Pose with a straight spine.

Mudra: Raise the right hand up as if taking an oath; fingers are together, straight, together and point up; the thumb rests against the hand. Place the left hand on the Heart Center, fingers together, pointing right, parallel to the ground, thumb relaxed. This is Sankalpa Asana, a posture of affirmation. On each inhale, with little movement, the right hand presses forward and the left hand presses inward against the Heart Center. The pressure of both hands is equal. On the exhale, release the pressure. Increase the pressure with each breath.

Breath: Breathe powerfully; keep the length of the inhale and the exhale equal.

Eye Focus: Focus the eyes on the Tip of the Nose.

Time: Continue for 11 minutes.

To End: Inhale, suspend the breath and press to the maximum, maintaining the pressure exhale. Maintain the posture and immediately begin Part 2.

Comments: The movement of the hands when pressing is no more than 5mm. The key is to balance the pressure of the arms.

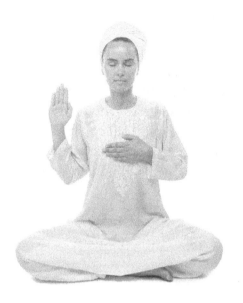 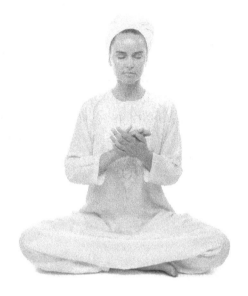

PART TWO

Remain in Easy Pose.

Mudra: Same as Part 1.

Breath: Light slow Long Deep Breathing, and later Breath of Fire.

Eye Focus: Close the eyes lightly.

Mantra: Waah Yantee (Version by Nirinjan Kaur is played)

WAAH YANTEE KAAR YANTEE,
JAGADOOTPATEE, AADAK IT WHAA-HAA,

BRAHMAADAY TRAYSHAA GUROO,
IT WHAA-HAY GUROO.

Time: Listen to the mantra for 6 minutes. Whisper the mantra strongly for 3 minutes. Then chant strongly for 2 minutes. The music stops. Maintain the posture with a strong fast Breath of Fire for 3 minutes.

To End: Inhale, hold for 15 seconds, exhale. Inhale, hold for 10 seconds, exhale. Inhale very deeply, hold tight for 40 seconds, exhale in Cannon Fire, extend the exhale for 7 seconds. Relax. Before beginning Part 3, shake the body.

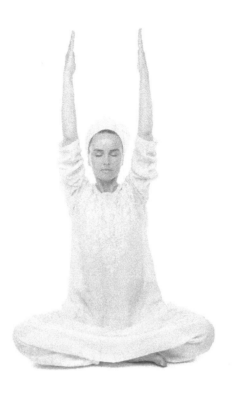

PART THREE

Remain in Easy Pose.

Mudra: Clap the hands in front of the body with palms horizontal, parallel to the ground. Flip the hands to alternate which is on top. The upper hand strikes the lower hand strongly.

Breath: Unspecified

Eye Focus: Unspecified

Mantra: *Punjabi Drums* is played to set the rhythm of the movement.

Time: Continue for 2 minutes.

To End: The music stops. Inhale deeply, suspend the breath, stretch the arms straight up and tighten the whole body, for 10 seconds. Cannon Fire exhale. Inhale deeply, stretch higher, hold for 15 seconds. Cannon Fire exhale. Inhale deeply once more, stretch even harder and hold for 25 seconds. Cannon Fire exhale and relax.

PRACTICAL TOOLS TO REMAIN IN ARADHANA

We need to be systematic to navigate the spaces of consciousness, create neural maps of those spaces, keep the relationship with ourselves, and foremost sustain this experience. Beyond practicing Kundalini Yoga, using pure devotion, we must also be receptive to the experience and study it as a science. Kundalini Yoga's techniques comprise an entire system that covers both physiological and psychological aspects of the body, which can restore the correct pranic flow through every meridian in the body. Our daily commitment to *Sadhana* with the different techniques to try, the fluctuating quality of the practice, the evolving development of consciousness, and the willingness to incorporate all of this into our daily life, requires a solid discipline to contain and consolidate the constant changes. The practitioner must create the habit of *Sadhana* by being present, in the wonder of innocence, and thus avoid the risk of repetitiveness.

Through the practice of *Sadhana*, we enter into a space in which we relate to ourselves and the universe, which rejects nothing. The *Sadaka*, one who follows this path, is like a bamboo tree exposed to and influenced by the environments – the wind, the sun, the rain, and the lunar phases while remaining firmly rooted in its own nature. He or she accepts and surrenders to the experience, moving and bending, becoming heavy or light in response to the environment, without trying to be something or find something, rather simply hungry to see through their essence, their life, and the world. Knowing their only desire is to improve their relation to Self, to use their potential fully. Without even searching for God, one is conscious that God is present in one's true Self. Thus, we play the game of union, accepting the boundaries of time and space. Through our perception, time exists to let things happen not all at once, and space exists, so things do not necessarily occur to us. The practitioner does not look for comfort or satisfaction. We seek reality and depth in the relations that we choose to engage in. We accept good and bad and are happy for any experience life throws at us. We do not practice to gain benefits. Our single intention is that the universe flow through us. We seek nothing from the known but rather receive what the Unknown gives us.

There is a big difference between the attitude to gain benefits and to accept what is already present, knowing we are part of the universal flow of prosperity. Both paths have a guiding principle, and they are different. The former is based on a dual vision, in which there is a separation between the universe and our potential. In contrast, the latter is based on a non-dual vision, in which there is no separation, nothing exists outside of ourselves, and every resource is already in potential, within us. The universe is our external representation, and we can comprehend it through ourselves.

We have seen that to understand ourselves and, thus, everything, it is vital to establish mental silence. Our growth is dependent on creating the right conditions to let the universal conscience flow within. Only then is it possible to improve our state of consciousness. Yoga, and Kundalini Yoga in particular, is not dual. It has a starting point and an objective but then moves from having a point of view to having none. Our attention and consciousness focus on a single point in order to merge with it. The result from practice and devotion to this sacred science is to find grace, even in the most ungraceful situation. Practice brings the virtue of non-reaction to the uncertainties of life. To reach this ability through *Aradhana* has always been the fuel of my personal *Sadhana*. In this state of perfect serenity, we accept our Self, retaining identity, grace, and peace within the events happening around us.

During the daily cleansing of the subconscious, as we observe minor concerns and worries rising to the surface, we learn to discern what to act upon and what to release. We learn to be in the totality of the experience. In our teachings, we know that as humans, we live in the need to confirm our existence, or we act in order to prove it. Through a rational process meant to identify ourselves, we tend to locate ourselves in relation to something, searching for a reference point to gain a feeling of ourselves. With the intuition and consciousness gained through our yoga practice, we can recognize and locate ourselves.

"As humans and healers, you have the ability to be in every place, the
question is: where are you not? You're always looking for a reference
point between time and space, and we use Yoga and Kundalini to break
this tendency. You are where you are. The only point of reference is you.
I know why I locate myself, because I AM, I AM, I AM. If I don't have a
reference, I can sit anywhere at every moment"
(Guru Dev Singh Khalsa).

After *Sadhana* educates us to be and act with rules and discipline, in *Aradhana* we need a different attitude. The goal is to improve our practice's quality, mental stability, and breadth of consciousness to maintain the depth of the experience. Change occurs in committed behavioral habits, physiological functions, and the flow of thoughts. We call this process transformation; actually, it is the emergence of who we are. There is no concept of gain or loss. A connection with a teacher's etheric body, the teachings themselves, and the Golden Chain support the process. Maintaining the quality of our practice and the balance between Shakti and Bhakti strengthen the connection. We have already learned that two and a half hours of practice in the early morning covers an entire day. Now we look at how practice can augment the awareness invoked in our morning *Sadhana* throughout the day. Around four in the afternoon, the alertness of our mental and physiological systems decreases. During this time, we make poor decisions and act impulsively. The support of yogic practices can lift the consciousness and bring back vitality for the last hours of the day. We can restore our vibratory frequency by repeating mantras, Bani or Shabd, our energetic levels through Pranayama, and replenish pranic flow in our bodies through a short kriya, like the "Sun Salutations".

In the evening before bedtime, to help release the day's stress and stimulate the brain's right hemisphere, bringing mental calmness, add a pranayama, a mantra, or a meditation. This routine improves the quality of sleep. With time, you will find that your *sadhana* governs every activity in the day.

Once we begin to practice daily *Sadhana*, it is surprising the changes that happen. What was vital is now obsolete; we gain energy. We sleep less, we produce more in less time, our relations improve, and we are healthy and efficient. We are no longer a product of our circumstances. We are consciously what we want to be.

Personally, my day has become rooted in the priority of my morning commitment *Sadhana*. Each day is divided into four and sometimes six parts, according to my needs. Sleeping comes first, requiring only four to six hours, the amount of time reduced by an evening meditation. When possible, I include several brief sessions of rest throughout the day, for example right after eating lunch. My personal practice, including the study of the techniques, includes 4 to 6 hours of the day, divided into *Sadhana*, afternoon yoga, reading Banis, and evening meditation. I consider going for a run or some other physical activity done with a meditative attitude as an integral part of my *Sadhana*. These activities help me to consolidate the meditative action by distributing the praana. It is conscious vitality in action. I dedicate 4 to 6 hours to work, for example organizing my activities and planning my financial state. The final 6 hours are dedicated to pure and simple Seva, which means any activity related to serving including serving family or people around you. By acknowledging the need for recreation, play and art, I try to allocate space to these whenever possible.

Self-Realization Kriya

June, 1996

Many religions do not focus on the Self but on a devotion to something greater and outside of you. The mantra *Humee Hum Brahm Hum* means We are God. We are asleep, and when we awaken, we see that we are divine. The Self has the negative and positive polarities and the neutral. The realm of the yogi is this neutral elevated Self.

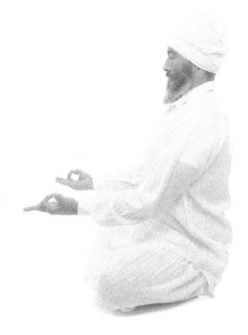

PART ONE

Sit in Easy Pose with a straight spine.

Mudra: Place the hands in Gyan Mudra, with the palms facing up and the fingers straight. Bend the elbows, keeping the forearms parallel to the ground and to each other. Stretch the upper arms forward until there is a weight in the shoulders.

Breath: Unspecified.

Eye Focus: Close the eyes and look at the chin.

Mantra: HUMEE HUM BRAHM HUM.

Chant using the tip of the tongue. (Version by Nirinjan Kaur is played)

Time: Continue for 7 minutes.

To End: Inhale and relax for 1 1/2 minutes.

Comments: When you create the weight on the shoulders, you work on the vagus nerve and energetically affect the 5th Chakra.

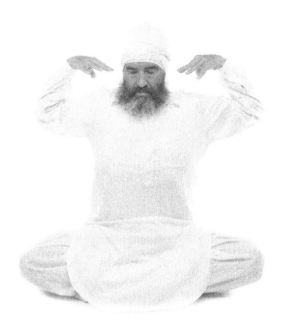

PART TWO

Remain in Easy Pose with a straight spine.

Mudra: Raise the arms out to the sides at shoulder level. Bend the elbows bringing the forearms slightly inward and up with the hands wider than and in front of the face at the level of the forehead. The palms face down with the fingers sharply bent down from the hands creating an angle. This posture puts pressure on the ribs at the level of the Heart Center. Hold and listen to the mantra.

Breath: Unspecified.

Eye Focus: Close the eyes and look at the chin.

Mantra: HUMEE HUM BRAHM HUM

Listen. (Version by Nirinjan Kaur is played)

Time: Continue for 3 minutes.

To End: Inhale, immediately drop the arms and relax. Stretch and move the shoulders and arms.

Comments: Kundalini Yoga is a science of angles and triangles. In this posture, feel them in your body and let them sustain your posture; do not use your muscular strength.

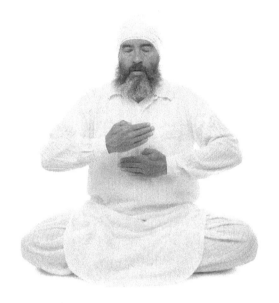

PART THREE

Remain in Easy Pose with a straight spine.

Mudra: Bend the elbows with the forearms parallel to the ground. Bring the hands in front of the Heart Center. Palms face the body. The left hand is close to the body and the right hand is 3" away from the back of the left hand. The forearms and hands move up and down, opposite each other in small, precise, quick movements. The upper arms do not move, the movement is from the elbows.

Breath: Unspecified.

Eye Focus: Close the eyes.

ATTITUDES, CONSCIOUSNESS, GOALS FOR PRACTICE

We have already introduced the *Mul Mantra*, a complete exploration of a human being's manifestation. We have spoken about our dormant potentiality and described some techniques to induce change. When we dare to embrace the vision described in the *Mul Mantra* and consistently practice *Sadhana*, we move towards *Aradhana*. The values and states of consciousness stated in the *Mul Mantra* are not distant goal. There are attainable. In *Aradhana*, the *Mul Mantra* is alive, a constant guide describing the universe and the relation between us as humans and everything else. Logic and reason move in the mandala of the most powerful sounds to express the Creator's essence along with his creation.

Ek Ong Kaar: To acknowledge and appreciate being part of the entire creation, holding the compelling vision of our connection to reality, full of accessible possibilities and resources. The opposites are in constant balance, holding the universe together. The Creator and the creature are thus the same thing.

Sat Naam: Observing our uniqueness as part of the creation and ourselves. Each creature with its own destiny: to live for this objective is the only chance to be happy and make others happy.

Kartaa Purakh: To acknowledge we are co-creators of the reality surrounding us and understand our relationship with that universe. By accepting ourselves in relation to the universe and committing to our destiny, we become one with our identity. We discover that we are the source and core of the whole vibratory effect we are experiencing. The place, situations and relations of our existence are the repercussion of our psyche's frequency, the effects of our thoughts and the consequences of our actions. Even if this responsibility seems heavy, it also gives rise to a sense of great honor. To feel the intimate relationship with the rest of creation provides a refreshing feeling of being sustained.

Nirbho: As co-creators of our lives, the intentions we have, the decisions we make, and the actions we take no longer come from our fear. The reactive impulse weakens, and what prevails is a neutral perception of what is real, allowing us to answer and act in alignment with our identity and destiny.

Nirvair: When fear is gone, we are not distracted by the perception of enemies or hostilities. The only danger can be ourselves if we do not stay true to our identity. Because we daily empty our subconscious, it no longer has a negative influence on our lives.

Akaal Moort: Free from the influence of a blocked subconscious, we live untethered beyond time and space. We live as if we were immortals, innocent, radiant, and magnificent. This is living in prosperity.

Ajoonee: In this flow, all effect of trauma from our birth and our parents' consciousness disappears.

Saibhung: We become conscious of the fact that no information can change us. We need nothing from the outside to excel because everything is within us.

Gurprasaad: We acknowledge that everything that we do or happens is a blessing, a gift that comes from the Infinite, and we are grateful for it.

Jap: The mind is in a state of prayerful gratitude, and we become a guide to others.

And concludes with: *Aad Such, Jugaad Such, Hai Bhee Such, Naanak Hosee Bhee Such.* True in the beginning, true throughout the ages, true even now, oh Naanak, truth shall ever be.

Progressing through the stages in the *Mul Mantra* leads to a radical change. As we have seen, Patanjali's eight limbs delineate the yogic aspects required to fine-tune the mind and experience reality. The *Mul Mantra* is an instrument to the manifestation of human potential. When practicing a kriya, if our attitude and consciousness include the *Mul Mantra* values, as well as the eight limbs of yoga, the actions we take will be the manifestation of God's will. Thus, the state of consciousness reached and the experience gained is without words; we can express it through our actions, tangible dharmic actions.

The spiritual path is almost beyond human comprehension, an indescribable conscious state that we know through experience. There is a guide, a technology, but no guarantee of success. The realization of this consciousness depends on the strength of one's will to walk this path and our willingness to sacrifice everything that gives an illusion of comfort and safety. We feel safe with what is known in our world and in what we believe is possible. Only after we identify what we truly want and commit to obtaining it will the impossible become possible. What the mind was unable to process before now looks possible. The discipline of the three stages of *Sadhana, Aradhana,* and *Prabhupati* creates the necessary conditions to negate presumptions and habits, resulting in an expansive consciousness. We reject reality because we are afraid to face something so vast. Then we deny it and remove it from our priorities. We become a non-priority. The practice of Kundalini Yoga that cleanses the subconscious aims to transform the lack of self-respect, self-esteem, and self-trust into strength and motivation.

Kriya for Endurance

September 14, 1992

In the Age of Aquarius, no matter what the circumstances, we need to know who we are in order to hold the balance. Whatever our actions or our words, there is always a polarity. One must prevail, *completely contained, content and conscious.*[4] What is required is endurance.

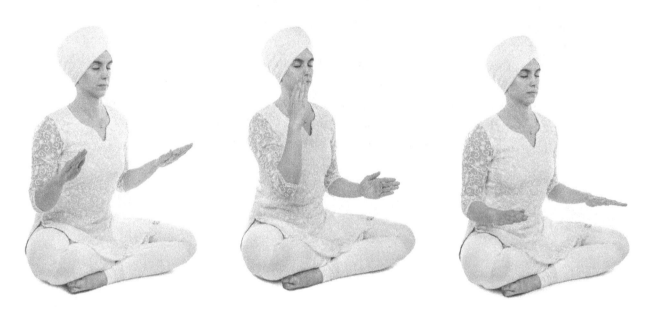

PART ONE

Sit in Easy Pose with a straight spine.

Mudra: With the upper arms by the body, bend the elbows, so that the bases of the hands are at shoulder level. The palms face forward and the fingers are relaxed. The movement is from the elbows and the forearms and hands move as a unit forward in the following sequence:

1) The hands move forward from the elbows in 3 quick continuous small movements.

2) For the 4th movement the right hand comes up with the forearm perpendicular to the ground and palm facing left, simultaneously the left forearm moves down parallel to the ground with the palm facing right.

3) Return to the starting position with both hands at the shoulder level palms facing forward.

4) All motions are a sharp jerk of the forearms with the wrists straight.

---

4 Yogi Bhajan, lecture January 4th, 1994

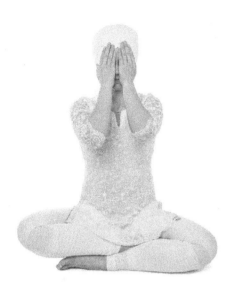
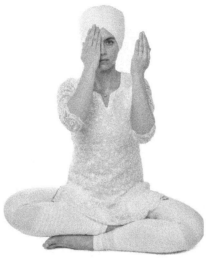
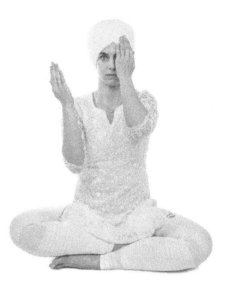

Breath: Not specified.

Eye Focus: Not specified.

Time: Continue for 11 minutes.

To End: Inhale deeply, hold the breath for 10 seconds and place the palms of both hands on the cheeks, fingers tightly cover the eyes.

Exhale. Repeat the breath two more times. Immediately begin Part 2.

Comments: This sequence of movements gives the nervous system a shock.

PART TWO

Remain in Easy Pose.

Mudra: Maintain the posture with the hands on the cheeks and fingers covering the eyes. Move both hands forward 18 inches away from the eyes and back. Move the hands quickly; touch the face gently.

Breath: Not specified.

Eye Focus: Keep the eyes open and look straight ahead.

Time: Continue for 4 minutes.

To End: Immediately begin Part 3.

Comments: Concentrate and hold the spine straight.

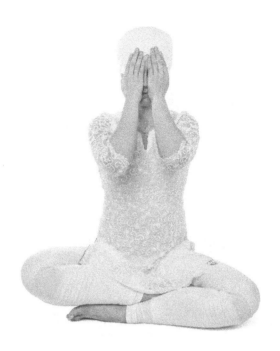

PART THREE

Remain in Easy Pose with a straight spine.

Mudra: Maintain the posture with the hands on the cheeks and fingers covering the eyes.

Breath: Not specified.

Eye Focus: Keep the eyes open, look straight through the darkness and see whatever you see. Study the colors.

Mantra: After 6 minutes, listen to *Five Religion Chant (Hallelujah)* by Mata Mandir Singh. Continue for 7 minutes.

Time: Total 13 minutes – 6 minutes in silence and 7 listening to the music.

To End: Maintain the posture. The music stops. Inhale deeply, and suspend the breath for 10 seconds. Exhale. Repeat two more times. Very slowly move the hands from the face, blink the eyes as fast as possible. Move the eyelids fast to bring circulation to the eyes. Continue for 30 seconds. Stretch and relax the body for 15 seconds. Immediately begin Part 4.

Comments: Self-healing starts by observing your own colors.

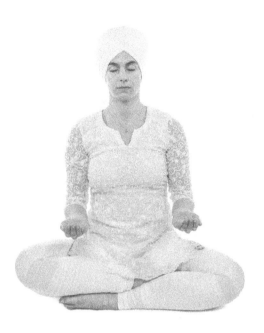
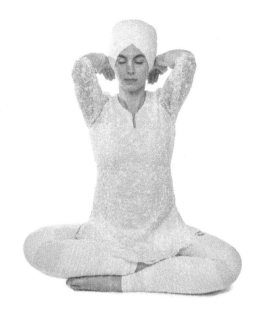

PART FOUR

Stand up and pick a partner. Greet each other, shake hands.

Mudra: Face your partner, hold hands if you wish. Dance anyway, as long as both feet are not on the ground at the same time.

Mantra: *Punjabi Drums* is played as rhythm for dancing.

Time: Continue for 11 minutes.

To End: Sit in Easy Pose with a straight spine. Upper arms are beside your body; bend the elbows with the forearms forward, parallel to the ground and each other. The hands are cupped with the palms up. Lift your hands up and over the shoulders as if quickly throwing water behind you. Create a strong jerking upward motion then quickly return to the starting position. Breath is unspecified. Continue for 40 seconds. Relax.

Comments: Dancing distributes the energy throughout the entire body.

APPLIED TECHNOLOGY FOR SELF-GUIDANCE

Life is the orbit traveled by the human psyche between space and time, the psyche that rotates around a vertical axis, just like the planets in our solar system. The rotation and the trajectory are determined by the human psyche, *karma* and *samskara*. The numerology of our birth date reflects the starting point – the longitude, latitude, time, and space. The orbit, the path, the endpoint, and the destiny can be calculated with these initial coordinates and the related push. The axis rotation is governed by who we are and our relationship with ourselves; the orbit is governed by how we preserve ourselves in life and how we act in our relationships. These two aspects need to be coordinated and coherent. Being only in line with the orbit might make us prosperous in the material side of life, but it will not necessarily make us happy. On the other hand, being in line with the axis rotation might bring harmony and happiness within our lives, but not necessarily prosperity in the material world. Time and space are the two challenges and opportunities given to the spiritual being in our human experience, as illustrated in the following diagram. [5]

---

[5] Based on an illustration in *Sadhana* Singh and Dunja Mladenic (2017), *Experiencing Leadership and Success.*

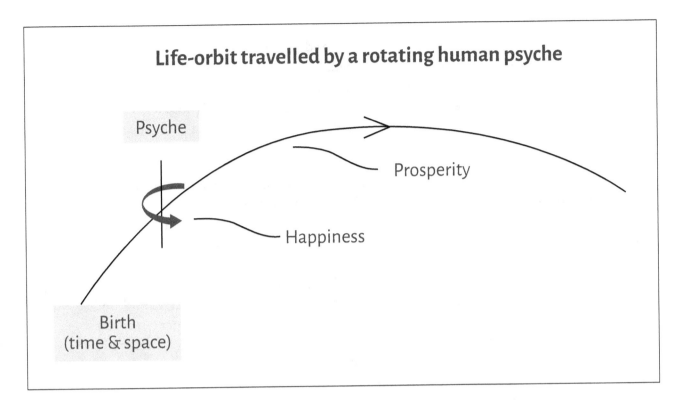

Life-orbit travelled by a rotating human psyche

To get up for *Sadhana* is victory over time and to do the practice is victory over space. In life, there are obstacles, challenges, and impossibilities limiting us from experiencing new possibilities. These obstacles, represented by different situations seen as external, reflect subconscious resistances existing before the initial trajectory. The external situation highlights the internal condition. Without an alternative to the initial trajectory, the endpoint will not change. Suffering, frustration, and sadness are consequences of the predictability and inevitability of the outcome. If we visualize a block as a square, we resolve the block using creative intelligence by dividing it into two triangles. When the diagonal energy cuts it precisely, the problem is not solved; it is dissolved. The polarities in life, the yes and no, the rights and wrongs, are revealed to the individual and dissolved. *Sadhana* is the context in which we train ourselves to have the conscious state diagonally penetrate the subconscious and dissolve the internal, the cause, thus resolving the external, the consequence.

Kundalini Yoga gives the lens to see under the surface, to grasp through our intuition the cause of what exists around and within us, and how to lift and remove the block. As we progress with our personal practice, the conscious mind sees these subconscious blocks. Often, the incongruence of our behavior compared to our true identity is the outcome of what we call "the hidden agenda", a small identity within us that makes us act for its needs, making us believe we are acting out of our own will. Over time, experiences we perceive as trauma or drama create this agenda. We lose the strength and power of our radiance and lose touch with reality. Assumptions and prejudices alter the reality of our experience. The senses are impoverished, and we become reactive. *Sadhana* is the space where we can observe and transcend these dynamics and lead us to the *Aradhana*. Living governed by the hidden agenda is living in ignorance. Having someone whom we trust to assist us in uncovering this agenda is of enormous help. Only when we become free from it can we relate to our true essence.

Intention and projection are two vital factors guiding us toward our destination and thus serving our consciousness. When we set a specific goal with the soul's intention, our entire being and intellect focus on it, in agreement to serve the intention. The seed of a thought, bloomed from the soul, released by the intellect, and held in purity to preserve its true nature, will align with the soul's intention. The mind uses its functions to serve the intention and start the manifestation. As we have seen, projection is the art of keeping the intention strong and projecting it forward and outward, filling the space, the environment, and the future. To understand our intention, we need to listen in silence. To follow it, we need courage and humility. To project it, we need consistency and authority. The intention determines the direction, the depth, and the vibration. When intention and projection align with the soul's will, the psyche's trajectory moves towards the destination. Finishing one's mission is our destination. The distance to reach that goal is life itself, and dharma can direct our life.

In *Sadhana*, if we observe that our intention comes from duality and fear, we decide not to identify with it and let it go. When we base our intention on our essence in neutrality, the projection serving it will be firm and gentle, flexible and focused. By living life consciously and intuitively, we return to wholeness; we are complete individuals. In *Aradhana*, by embracing the polarities, a genuine reverence for ourselves surfaces, and together with the power of projection, we can realize everything. We understand there is nothing but our Self. Everything we encounter in life, both people and situations, are there because we permit them to be present. The space we give them in our consciousness creates the conditions for them to manifest, and the reaction to their presence blocks our neutrality to act decisively.

There are three levels of truth: *personal, circumstantial, and infinite.* In our spiritual practice, we learn to recognize and trust the infinite truth and live according to its unseen laws. If we has not yet gained the maturity to live in the infinite truth, let personal truth, not the circumstances decide how we act. The practice of Kundalini Yoga leads us to expand our perception and transcend circumstances to endure the unendurable with grace.[6]

---

[6] Yogi Bhajan, lecture May 13th, 1985

Kriya to Balance Your Electromagnetic Field and Your Psyche

September 18, 1996

When you have command of your actions, the wave of your emotions no longer rules you. In *Jaapji Sahib*, Guru Nanak expresses the adage *you reap what you sow* with the following words:

"Karmee Aapo aapnee, kay nerai kay door."
"According to their own actions, some are drawn closer, and some are driven farther away."

Our actions determine everything. This brings us back to discipline of clearing the subconscious so that we act from our purity, not from our pain and anger.

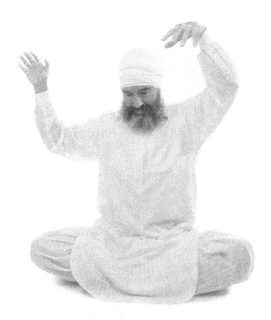

PART ONE

Sit in Easy Pose with a straight spine.

Mudra: Raise the arms out to the sides with the upper arms shoulder height. Bend the elbows, so that the forearms face straight ahead and are raised 45 degrees; the hands and fingers are relaxed and the wrists are straight and locked. From the elbows, shake the forearms and hands powerfully and quickly; the force will shake the entire body. The movement is like a vibration and is so strong that the entire spine from lower back to the neck moves.

Breath: Not specified.

Eye Focus: Not specified.

Time: Continue for 6 minutes. Immediately begin Part 2.

Comments: Use your inner anger to fuel the motion. The goal is to move so hard that you get out of breath.

229

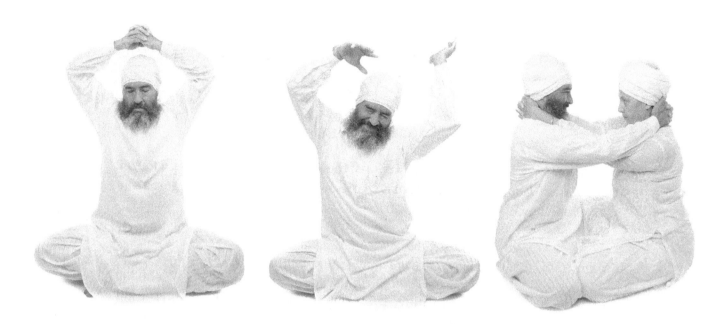

PART TWO

Remain in Easy Pose with a straight spine.

Mudra: Interlace the fingers over the head, palms facing down, creating an arc with the arms. Pull the hands apart without releasing them. Pull with as much force as possible.

Breath: Breathe normally.

Eye Focus: Not specified.

Time: Continue for 1 minute.

To End: Inhale deeply, hold tight and squeeze the spine upward for 10 seconds, cannon fire exhale. Repeat 2 more times. Relax. Then move your elbows, wrists, fingers and shoulders. Continue for 1 minute. Immediately begin Part 3.

Comments: The navel is automatically pulled in.

PART THREE

Remain in Easy Pose.

Mudra: Dance the body, move every part of the body as if in ecstasy. Feel free, do not be concerned with how you look, just dance your subtle body, absolutely dance the way you want to dance.

Breath: Not specified.

Eye Focus: Not specified.

Time: Continue for 2 minutes.

To End: If you are practicing with others, sit face to face with a partner. Lock the hands behind the neck of the partner and look straight into each other's eyes. Inhale; suspend the breath, pull, and resist as hard as possible for 10 seconds. Exhale. Repeat two more times, on the last breath suspend for 15 seconds. If you are practicing alone, interlace your fingers and place them on the back of the neck, pull forward with the hands as you resist with the head and neck. Relax.

From Dream to Reality

The goal of a spiritual practice is to have a clear and vast mind that can comprehend and accept the polarity game and the fluctuations of life, and thus, we can calibrate our existence on our soul's will in relation to reality. We see this concept in the scriptures: *"Mann vidh channan vekiya"* meaning to penetrate through the mind and make a hole in it to gain the infinite vision of reality.[7] Without this, we live hidden and defensive, closed to the inner voice, missing the experiences that lead to transformation. This opening is impossible when the mind is so dense, filled with preconceived concepts and unconscious patterns. For this reason, we benefit when we periodically shift from our routine to be awake and remember the infinite capacities of the mind and the braveness of the soul.

Each Kundalini Yoga practitioner finds certain kriyas and meditations most beneficial for them and uses them as an anchor in their daily *sadhana*. For me personally, the Praan Shashtar Kriya and the Sat Siri Kriya serve this function. They have been a constant, unchanging presence in my *sadhana* for years, while other kriyas and meditations alternate in cycles from forty to a thousand days. These two kriyas are intense and require time to build up the practice and internalize the effects gradually. It took me just under a year to practice them adequately and years to comprehend their dynamics and effects. Today, I do not feel like I am an expert, but rather an honest practitioner who continues to discover more effects. Yogi Bhajan recommended a daily practice with the

---

[7] Yogi Bhajan, Los Angeles lecture, March 8th, 1983

recitation of *Japji Sahib* and Sat Kriya. They have a complementary action. Together, they train the pranic body, stimulate the subtle body and reinforce the nervous system. The recitation of *Japji Sahib* is within Praan Shashtar Kriya, and Sat Siri Kriya is a variation of Sat Kriya.

In Praan Shashtar Kriya, we recite *Japji Sahib* in Platform Pose. The sound wave vibration (*Nada Brahman*) in this specific posture aids the sound's resonance in the *Sushumna* channel and the flow through the other *nadis*. The challenge lies in allowing this process while holding the challenging posture. The body fights to keep itself in the asana, the breath becomes shallow, the lower back may hurt, and we speak faster and cut our words short. We need time and patience to relax in this posture, to feel and open to the sound current. As with all practices, the experience varies according to the attitude we have during the practice. If we struggle using force, we are fighting an impossible battle and will uselessly suffer without obtaining the desired effect. On the other hand, if we have an attitude of devotion and humility, we reap unexpected benefits with determination and consistency. In other words, the key to this practice is not physical strength. In Sat Siri Kriya, instead of Rock Pose – the stable seated position we usually use in Sat Kriya –, the starting posture is squatting on the balls of the feet with the heels together – a less grounded posture. To maintain balance requires holding a relaxed tension. The only controlled movement in this position's stillness is the pull and release of the navel. The support in both kriyas is silence and shuniya. Anything else results in a struggle.

Another practice suggested – this one by Guru Dev Singh – is the repetition for one hour of the mantra *Guroo Guroo Whaa-hay Guroo Guroo Raam Daas Guroo* beginning at three in the morning. He said, "Do me a favor, practice this meditation". This practice assists the kundalini in rising and strengthens our connection with the Golden Chain. The magic and challenge of this meditation lie in its simplicity, and the early morning time. The belief is that this is the best time to connect with the presence of Guru Ram Das. A constant dedication to this practice requires a very determined effort. However, the consciousness state attained is worth the sacrifice. The meditation starting at 3:00 am concludes at 4:00 am. In the *Amrit Vela*, we may choose to continue our *sadhana* or be tempted to go back to bed. After an hour of meditation, the subconscious is fully open, and going back to sleep may result in an uncontrolled release of the subconscious, possibly countering the benefits of the previous meditation. Thus, if going back to sleep, it is recommended to nap for no more than 20 minutes, followed by a shortened *Sadhana* to reset the psyche and the magnetic field. This simple meditation, working on subconscious obstructions and opening the chakras, impacts our physical and emotional health. Just once in your life, practice it daily for 120 days.

If you want to invest some time to know your mind in a systematic and educational way, practice each of the meditations in the book, *The Mind*.[8] Then, this information becomes a concrete experience, rather than simply intellectual information. You will literally create in your mind a map of the interactions and combinations of the functional and impersonal minds and the *gunas*. To experience each mental state opens new possibilities. What, at first, seems to be a complex system composed of incomprehensible concepts becomes understandable by experiencing each state in meditation. We can recognize these qualities in our Self and others, and most of all, we become aware of how to restore a balance.

Studying these meditations systematically is very valuable for every human being, especially those who teach Kundalini Yoga. If you practice the meditations for each of the nine aspects for forty days, you will gain a basic understanding of the mind in a little less than a year. After that, to deepen your understanding further, you may study the three projections of each aspect. If you decide to practice the meditations for the aspects and the projections, it will require approximately three years to complete.

A final recommendation for a personal practice is *Sukhmani Sahib's* recitation, a text of the Sikh tradition that has the unique quality to keep the consciousness open and elevated during the entire day. The text has twenty-four chapters (*ashtapadi*) representing the twenty-four hours of the day. One can read it any time during the day or divide it into sections to read throughout the day. If we choose to read it at once, the best time is at the start of the day. The vibration persists throughout the day, easing life's challenges. If dividing it into sections, there are two preferred methods: reading three *ashtapadi* eight times a day (every 3 hours) or reading eight *ashtapadi* three times a day (every 8 hours).

The choice of reading every three hours is based on an ancient concept of time and energy, which divides the day into eight segments because changes in attitudes, rhythms, and tendencies occur every three hours. During these intervals, the radiance, expansion, and frequency of the magnetic field changes. This corresponds with the breath's change from one nostril to the other, varying our sensibility, comprehension, and projection. The sound current from the recitation of *Sukhmani Sahib* at these intervals is said to support these natural fluctuations. The choice of reading eight *ashtapadi* three time, although no

---

[8] Gurucharan Singh Khalsa and Yogi Bhajan, The Mind – Its Projections and Multiple Facets, Published by Kundalini Research Institute, New Mexico, 1998.

longer supporting the natural cycles, attends to three basic times in our day – awakening when we reset the physical, mental and energetic functions, the shadow zone at four in the afternoon, when the psychophysical state makes us prone to unwise choices, and preparing for sleep when we release the concerns of the day, prepare for a regenerative sleep and set the conditions for a successful day ahead. No matter how and when we read it. Over time, when our neutrality falters in face of problems and worries, the sound current of *Sukhmani* fills the mind, so neutrality prevails.

Sukhmani Sahib does not speak about rituals, discipline, diet, or asceticism. Instead, it evokes and explains one of the highest states of yogic consciousness, *Simran*, the ability to be in a constant meditative state. *Sukhmani* is an extraordinary poetic work designed to spiritually elevate those who read and listen to its sound and its teachings with devotion. Letting it come through our hearts will make pain, illnesses, and duality disappear. By understanding and practicing its teachings, the human life is instantly saved and directed towards its destiny, every action is full of virtue, and one's words flow like nectar.

This prayer, given by Guru Arjan is a tool to successfully overcome the dark age of Kali Yuga (the current age known as the Iron Age) and to free us from the cycle of birth, death, and rebirth. It also discusses practical aspects of life. Those who read it with devotion claim it brings prosperity and material richness, improves relationships, grants the ability to heal others and the self, and to experience harmony and peace within themselves and with others

.

Praan Shashtra Kriya

June 26, 1990

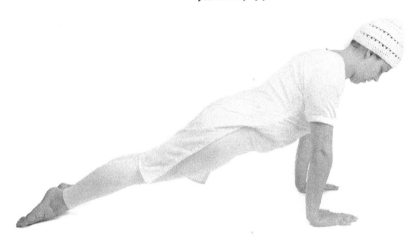

Posture: Front Platform Pose: Begin on the hands and knees. Place the palms on the ground, shoulder width apart and under the shoulders, arms straight. Stretch both legs back, tops of the feet on the ground creating a straight line from the top of the head to the toes. Author's Note: If you are unable to hold the posture, rest, when needed or modify by lightly resting the knees on the ground, while maintaining a straight line from the knees through the neck.

Breath: Not specified.

Eye Focus: Not specified. Eyes may be open if you are reading the text.

Mantra: Read Japji Sahib out loud.

Time: One recitation of Japji Sahib approximately 25 minutes.

Comments: Never practice this kriya alone. Someone must be with you to keep you grounded. The first two parts of this kriya build up endurance and stamina in the nervous system. When you perfect Japji in this pose, you gain control over your praana.

Sat Siri Kriya

June 26, 1990

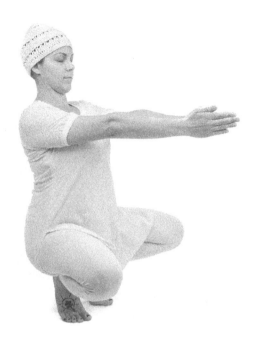

Posture: Frog Pose Variation: With the heels together and feet at a 45 degrees angle, squat down and balance on the balls of the feet. Keep the spine straight and as upright as possible. Raise the arms parallel to the ground, straight in front of the body. Press the palms together, keep the elbows straight and fingers point straight forward.

Breath: Not specified.

Eye Focus: Look at the Tip of the Nose.

Mantra: SAT NAAM

Chant as done in Sat Kriya.

Time: Not specified.

Author's Note: It best not to interrupt the steady chanting of Sat Naam. If you are unable to maintain the posture, modify by letting the heels be on the ground or consider coming out of the squat and standing.

Meditation to Open the Sushumna

November 6, 1985

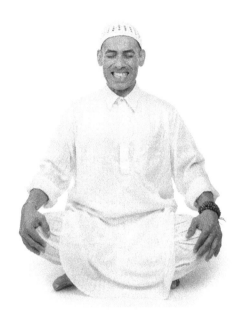 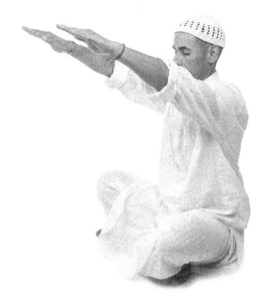

PART ONE

Sit in Easy Pose with a straight spine.

Mudra: Hands relaxed. Shape your mouth into a "Leo Smile, the smile of the lion". Bring the front teeth together with a small space between them, tighten the lips and pull back the corners of the mouth to show the teeth.

Breath: Cannon Breath from the Navel Point; inhale and exhale powerfully through the teeth.

Eye Focus: Not specified.

Time: Continue for 5 minutes. Immediately begin Part 2.

PART TWO

Mudra: Remain in Easy Pose. Raise the arms straight forward and up to 60 degrees. Elbows straight, fingers together, and palms face down.

Breath: Not specified.

Eye Focus: Eyes are closed.

Visualization: Visualize being at the edge of an infinite body of water just about to dive in, on the edge of letting go.

Time: Continue for 3 minutes. Immediately begin Part 3.

Comments: The power is in being in the mental state of readiness to leap, transmuting the energy of the lower triangle to find the clarity within the purity.

PART THREE

Mudra: Maintain the posture.

Breath: Not specified.

Eye Focus: Eyes remain closed.

Visualization: Visualize releasing and diving into the water. Dive deep through the blue layers, through Infinity and touch the bottom.

Time: Continue for 1 minute.

To End: Inhale deeply, suspend the breath and relax out of the posture. Suspend the inbreath up to 1 minute while you visualize the body floating back up through the water. See the surface of the water getting closer faster as the breath suspension comes near its end. Feel the head close to the surface. Breaking through exhale. Relax.

Kriya to Create Electromagnetic Field to Expand the Self

June 4, 1986

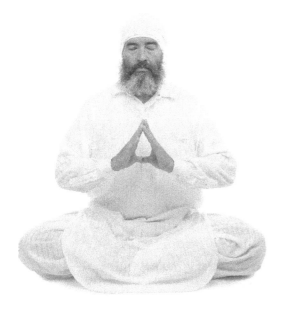

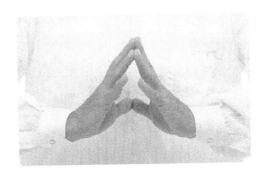

PART ONE

Sit in Easy Pose with a straight spine.

Posture: Bring the elbows out to the sides, forearms parallel to the ground, hands in front of the Heart Center. Place the pads of the Jupiter Fingers (index fingers), Saturn Fingers (middle fingers), Sun Fingers (ring fingers) and the thumbs together, Mercury Fingers (pinky fingers) and palms do not touch, fingers are straight and point up, thumbs point toward the body.

Breath: Breathe with the music in the following rhythm: Inhale deep and exhale completely with each repetition of "Waa-Hay Guroo", hold the breath out until the next repetition of Waa-Hay Guroo. If the music is not available, inhale for 4 seconds, exhale for 4 seconds, suspend the breath out for 7 seconds. Continue this breath pattern.

Eye Focus: Tip of the Nose.

Mantra: Originally taught with *I am Thine* by Livtar Singh.

Time: Continue for 12 minutes

To End: Relax the breath and the posture.

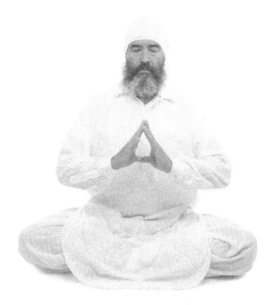

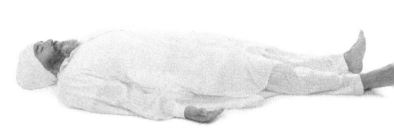

PART TWO

Remain in Easy Pose.

Posture: Come into the same posture as Part One.

Breath: Breathe with the music in the following rhythm: Breath of Fire with each repetition of the chorus ("Walking up the mountain..."), inhale deeply at the end of the chorus and suspend the breath for the duration of the verse. Repeat Breath of Fire with the chorus.

Eye Focus: Unspecified.

Mantra: Originally taught with *Walking up the Mountain* by Gurudass Singh.

Time: Continue for 8 minutes. Immediately begin the next part.

PART THREE

Posture: Come lying on your back and relax completely.

Mantra: Play light, sweet music.

Time: Continue 13 minutes.

To End: Remain on the back and roll the feet and hands for 20 seconds. Practice Cat Stretch for 30 seconds. Immediately begin the next part.

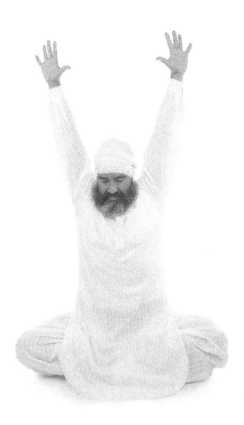

PART FOUR

Sit in Easy Pose with a straight spine.

Posture: Move the arms, shoulders, spine, the entire body. Stretch every part of the body.

Breath: Unspecified.

Eye Focus: Unspecified.

Mantra: Continue music from Part Three.

Time: Continue for 3 minutes. Immediately begin the next part.

PART FIVE

Remain in Easy Pose with a straight spine.

Mantra: *Sing Song of the Khalsa*, version by Gurudass Singh and Gurudass Kaur was played in class.

Time: Continue for 7 minutes.

To End: Relax.

Comments: To have the maximum effect from this kriya, the morning after you practice, have 12 ounces of prune juice as your breakfast. This will relax and bring new energy to your mental capacity.

I Am My Grace Meditation

April 13, 2000

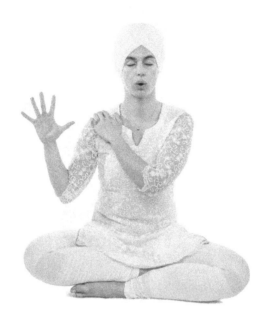

Sit in Easy pose with a straight spine.

Mudra: Place the left hand on the top of the right shoulder, palm flat, fingers relaxed, elbow relaxed. The right elbow is relaxed at the side. Raise the right hand by the right shoulder, like taking an oath, fingers straight, palm forward.

Breath: Breathe powerfully through an 'O' mouth. Inhale in three strokes, exhale in one stroke.

Eye Focus: The eyes are closed.

Time: Continue for 11 minutes.

To End: Inhale deeply, suspend the breath for 15 seconds, raise both hands up and stretch your spine up as much as possible. Exhale. Keep the arms up, inhale, suspend for 15 seconds. Exhale. Inhale deeply, suspend the breath for 15 seconds, stretch up and spread the fingers wide, make them like steel. Cannon Fire exhale, and relax.

Comments: When doing this as a daily personal practice, alternate the arms (reverse the posture) daily with the same breath pattern.

Guidance of the Soul Meditation

July 22, 1996

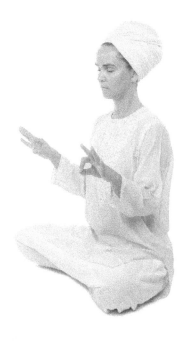
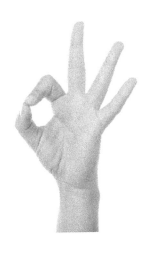

Sit in Easy Pose with a straight spine.

Mudra: The hands are in Gyan Mudra. The other fingers are straight and spread as wide apart as possible. The upper arms and elbows press into the rib cage. The forearms are shoulder width apart, tilted forward 45 degrees from the shoulders. On each repetition of Har (or every second), keeping the elbows tight to the ribs, the forearms strongly jerk back and up to just in front of the shoulders and immediately relax back to the starting position at 45 degree forward and down. The movement is so strong that the entire body jumps off the ground with the movement of the forearms.

Breath: Not specified.

Eye Focus: Not specified.

Mantra: The *Tantric Har* creates the rhythm of the movement (1 per second). It is not chanted.

Time: Continue 11 minutes.

Comments: This kriya is known as *Gyan Sudhaa Simran Kriya*. It is not an easy practice. The goal of the meditation is to enter the state of *Simran*. You live in constant meditation, no matter what you are doing. Then the soul radiates and takes us beyond the senses.

In *Simran*, a state of consciousness without ego, we learn not to fear nobility. This is what we have come to learn; it is the goal of human existence.

Ungali Praanayam Meditation

May 1, 1975

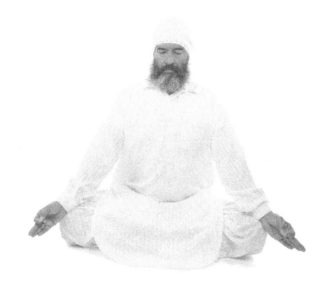

Sit in Easy Pose with a straight spine.

Mudra: Place the hands in Gyan Mudra on the knees, elbows straight.

Breath: Inhale in 15 equal segments through the nose. Exhale in 15 equal segments through the nose.

Eye Focus: Not specified.

Mantra: Mentally vibrate the Panj Shabd with the breath as follows:

Inhale: SAA, SAA, SAA, SAA, SAA, SAA, SAA, SAA, SAA, SAA, SAA, SAA, SAA, SAA, SAA

Exhale: TAA, TAA, TAA, TAA, TAA, TAA, TAA, TAA, TAA, TAA, TAA, TAA, TAA, TAA, TAA

Inhale: NAA, NAA, NAA, NAA, NAA, NAA, NAA, NAA, NAA, NAA, NAA, NAA, NAA, NAA, NAA

Exhale: MAA, MAA, MAA, MAA, MAA, MAA, MAA, MAA, MAA, MAA, MAA, MAA, MAA, MAA, MAA

One cycle of the mantra takes about 30 seconds.

Time: Continue for 3 minutes. Add 1 minute per day, gradually build up to a maximum of 31 minutes.

To End: Inhale, exhale and relax. Enjoy.

Sahaj Yoga Meditation

January 12, 1976

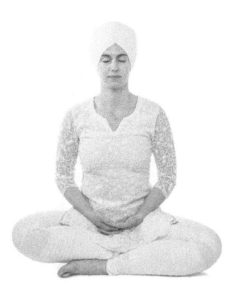

Sit in easy pose with a straight spine.

Mudra: Place your hands in your lap, right hand resting in the left hand with the thumbs gently touching.

Breath: Long Deep Breath.

Eye Focus: The eyes are 9/10th closed.

Visualization: As you inhale, mentally travel along the spine from the tailbone to the top of the head and down to the Tip of the Nose. As you exhale, mentally travel from the Tip of the Nose to the top of the head and down the spine to the tailbone. Envision a white light moving along the spine as the breath travels up and down.

Mantra: On the inhale, mentally chant MAHAAN KAAL.

On the exhale, mentally chant KAAL KA.

Time: Continue for 11 minutes.

To End: Inhale, raise the arms up over the head and vigorously shake your hands. Exhale and relax. Inhale, stretch the arms up once again, and shake the hands rapidly. Exhale and relax.

Comments: Mahan Kal means the great flow of being and Kal Ka, the flow of eternal power (the Kundalini). It is said that this meditation was practiced by Guru Gobind Singh (the Tenth Sikh Master) three hundred years ago. Any person can raise their level of consciousness with this meditation.

PRABHUPATI

Merging with our Self

In *Sadhana*, there is the urge to be with the divine lover, the One within us. Driven by love and the desire for belonging, we commit to being the bride of the Beloved. The wedding happens in *Aradhana*, with a sacred commitment, and we experience the joys and challenges to maintain the desired union. In *Prabhupati*, we face two polarities, attraction and repulsion, and see them as two sides of the same coin. They are complementary and act as one. Radiance prevails when there is an absence of doubt, providing certainty of the union. The polarities, in neutrality, no longer conflict; they are together in the unknown. *Purusha*, transcending the challenges of time and space, conquers the creativity of creation, *Prakriti*, with all the layers of Maya, and acknowledges the Creator in everything.

Thus, human beings go from their limited, finite ego identification to identifying with the infinite truth, *Sat Naam*. Their finite and infinite natures unite in consciousness. If we ignore or, in judgment, reject the union of the opposites living paradoxically within, we polarize our understanding based on what the mind sees as right or wrong. In addition to the enormous energy required to contain this polarization, we feel the pain of being incomplete, unsatisfied, and unreal. On the other hand, if we recognize this oneness, we feel complete within and a part of everything, a co-creator of our life and destiny.

Sadhana, Aradhana, and *Prabhupati* are the creative disciplinary functions that harmonize the polarities within us. Through neutrality, they allow us to see our true Self and express it through actions. Affecting the creation with our uniqueness confirms the indispensable role we have in the world. When we judge others or ourselves without seeing the Creator within, we cause our own suffering. We diminish ourselves, feeling guilty that we are broken, and look for what we perceive we lack outside of ourselves. This becomes a never-ending pursuit because there is nothing outside. Everything is within us. All we need to change is our relationship with our inner universe. This will improve our relationships with others and ourselves, and we will be in harmony with the universal will. Each of us is a creation of God. We feel God within us and in others, as well as in nature.

To experience the Creator, who is pure creativity, is thus a creative process. Like the colors on a painter's palette, creativity consists of differences, opposites, and contrasts. Similarly, our inner being is complete and perfect in itself, in its oneness, and at the same time, the chaos in us, as in the universe, is our potential creativity. The variant conditions lead to changes in the structure, both short and long term. This is true for the universe and our microcosmic selves and their continuous interaction and reciprocal influence. *Sadhana*, *Aradhana*, and *Prabhupati*, through the application of the technology of Kundalini Yoga, induce small changes in the psyche, subtle changes in the consciousness, moderate alterations of the energetic levels, imperceptible differences in the neuronal connections, producing tangible expansion on a perceptional, cognitive and executive level.

The state of *Prabhupati* implies a deep experiential understanding of the polarities within us: the light and the dark, the tendencies and opposing resistances, the fantasies and rationalities, the intuitive insights and impulses. Then, further, use and manage this understanding to become the authors of the best and most complete expression of ourselves, rather than a victim of circumstances. With self-knowledge of our totality and the universal creative essence, we are experts of creation itself. In our earlier analogy of *Prabhupati* being the marriage, the merger is such that the bride-to-be is not just the bride of God but also the master of God. The state of *Prabhupati* is mastery of the Self; what we say, intend and do, affects the universal psyche.

Based on the root of the word, the original purpose of religion is similar to *Prabhupati*. The word religion comes from *re* – frequency and cadence and, *ligere–* choice, *re-ligere* – to look attentively, to unify. Religion is thus the science of reality investigating our own origins and the choice whether to reunify or stay separated. This also is the foundation and purpose of yoga. Yoga is the means to reach clarity with reality and the conscious presence to decide what to be. In religion, God is the object of the research. If we are the creature of the creator's creation, we are God, and in *Prabhupati* we merge with ourselves.

The Mastery of The Self

The word mastery comes from the root *magis*, meaning 'great', reinforced by *ter*, giving it the sense of 'greatest.' Mastery in our case does not imply that we are superior to others. Rather, we have overcome the given conditions to embrace totality and live our creative potential fully. Our identity is divinity – in other words, union, not division. It starts with finding and being ourselves in order to understand our role in the universe. Functioning from our essence, we ignore the ego-self and dedicate ourselves to serve. With increased experience and competency, we gain mastery. Therefore, beyond the subconscious mind's dynamics of gain and loss, we retain and manifest our intention without changes in its essence. The Self assigns itself; the Self gives itself in service, consistent with its purpose. When it is possible to achieve this, we can assist others. That is how to become a master.

Great discipline is required to overcome the internal conflicts resulting in polarization and, instead, find a solution to the given challenges through elevation, not polarization. With self-awareness, it is possible to observe ourselves and overcome reactive behavior and other behavior patterns that lead to repetitive mistakes. In the previous sections, we discussed these dynamics in depth. They are woven into the psychic subconscious. They thrive in the perceptive memories of the first eleven years of life. They form a long list of demands, needs, and expectations, building hidden agendas and hidden, reactive personalities. When these masked subconscious identities take hold, we are not masters. Instead, we are victims of a circumstantial hidden reality that has little to do with our authentic being and the reality of the moment.

Nonetheless, these tendencies seem unstoppable and unmanageable for us because they seem to be the only viable option. The horizon loses its vastness; our subconscious convinces the conscious mind that this is the only way, justifying it with stories. At this time, we must stay alert, have a kind heart and a compassionate mind. When the subconscious vetoes the impossible, we consciously do the impossible and bring our heart in our mind and our mind in our heart to be and act with the mind's heart and the heart's wisdom. Together in this union, we become whole and act rather than react to the circumstance.

We prove that we are masters when we act consciously with excellence, overcoming the subconscious tendency to see a given situation as impossible— no longer sabotaging the Self. There is no repression, control, or resistance, but instead consciously being and letting our spirit prevail. This alone is not enough. When we no longer react subconsciously, we need to gather our resources and mental and perceptive functions to manage the circumstances while keeping the integrity and altitude. The gradual development through *Sadhana, Aradhana,* and *Prabhupati* leads in time to an intuitive and analytical understanding of how our intentions, words, and actions cause the desired consequences. In creation, there is a creative process regulating the dynamics of success. To create what we sincerely want, showing our essence and uniqueness, we first must recognize and then reject the subconscious "destructive" creative process. Once this mastery is integrated, we can excel in any situation. The creative process is thus creativity itself. We need to understand this in both directions, from intention and conception to manifestation and vice versa, from cause to consequence and consequence to cause.

MIRAGE OR MASTERY

The ability to excel and realize our intentions is proportional to how much influence the subconscious mind has over us. This is the simple truth. The power of the psychic subconscious contents comes from complex stories and associations reinforcing strong beliefs and habits that can confuse the reality in front of us. Subconscious agendas transform everything we perceive, remember or imagine. Therefore, it is able to confuse us so much that we might think that we have eluded it and wrongly think we are free from its power, while it continues to rule our lives. Discrimination is therefore vital in order to recognize what is real from what is not.

If nothing activates them, subconscious memories, their tendencies and habits may remain dormant for a long time. The opposite virtue can suppress a reactive compulsion, until the right catalyst activates it. Sometimes, one pattern represses others that are neither dissolved nor mastered, but instead temporarily eclipsed. Even if we are conscious of the dynamics, we may pretend to others and ourselves that we are unrestrained by them. Our motivation must be strong, as love fuels this process. We learn from the experience of people who in the past were brave enough to make this spiritual journey, that it is possible to live without limit in a limited condition. The common element in each unique spiritual journey is love.

The incentive to start on our self-exploration is the lack of love, often expressed as the desire to be loved, to belong, and be one. The gradual experience of love, the slight taste of love for oneself, life, and others are rays of light that keep us going. Love transforms demoting habits and vices into promoting habits and virtues, making them strengths in their own uniqueness. Like other forms of yoga, Kundalini Yoga aims to make conscious automatic physiological functions, such as breath and heartbeat, and the mechanical ones, such as posture, movement, and choice of thoughts and actions. This includes conscious awareness as the guiding light to perceive truth within subconscious thoughts and patterns. With the meditative mind, we evaluate every discernment using wisdom and intuition. Those who have mastery are full of love, illuminated thoughts, magnetic words, surprising presence, and unpredictable actions. We cannot judge mastery merely from actions but rather the motivation and the process behind the actions.

Integrity in the Process

The process of mastery is the art of conscious intervention in our own lives and active participation in the co-creation of our personal reality, both the universal and the circumstantial. The neutral and intuitive mind, constantly in a meditative state, must project our reality while interacting with our situation's totality. After first becoming conscious of the subconscious habits, we need to restructure and elevate them to convey our essence. When the subconscious is in line with consciousness in terms of contents and vibratory frequency, external events do not disturb our intent; this is mastery. When the internal intention and the external projection have the same objective, we gain our perceptive and creative power. Knowing ourselves, we consciously alternate between contraction and expansion rather than unconsciously polarizing.

How can one keep our intentions during the long process of becoming? What might help us make the right decisions? What is our compass to show us the right direction and maintain it without getting lost? At some point, we reach a crossroad, the choice between a life spent trying to achieve what we think might satisfy us or a life lived with love and joy. This is the difference between normalcy and spirituality, dreaming of happiness and being happy, between taking and giving, scarcity and abundance, doubt and trust.

At some time in our life, we felt insecure and a lack of belonging and love. We tried to fill that emptiness and ease the pain by looking outside to things, people, or status but remained in distress. When we allow ourselves to feel the discomfort and live with it, we find satisfaction from a personal relationship with our Self, which extends to others and the environment. The yogi understands this second way; the goal of all yoga is to achieve oneness. The yogi becomes calm, meditates, and senses the universe's flow and its role within the creation. In other words, conscious of themselves and their uniqueness, they intuitively grasp where, when, and how to act. The universe lovingly offers the chance to participate in universal creativity. The yogi understands that the loving action is to know thyself. Who you are, not what you want, must be the core around which life rotates.

We acknowledge that most of our life is spent running after what we want, believing that once this is obtained, we will be happy. Often this search is exhausting and creates unwanted consequences, resulting in more suffering. The universe wants us to have time and space simply to be ourselves. To do this, we must redefine our primary need from want to have to want to be. Thus, in the first stage of this change, we own ourselves. To be oneself is not enough. In the second stage, we learn to be without the being, without the self. We offer ourselves to serve others and the universe through our uniqueness. We sustain our new self through service, for only through giving our true Self is it possible to be oneself. If we really want to become masters of ourselves, we need to offer our selves.

History teaches us that nobody has become a master because they wanted it, but because they obeyed and served. They obeyed their higher selves and served by giving their uniqueness, committed to something greater than their individuality. A humble person is a potential master, taming the limited ego, seeing the vastness in the teachings, and trusting their higher Self in devotion to the teachings. Those who want to become masters may reach that status, while those who serve not only reach the status but also the consciousness of a master and leave a great legacy. The difference lies in whether the Infinite's strength dwells within. When it does, a master's presence communicates without words.

The challenges we attract in being and expressing ourselves, as complex as they might be, are appropriate in their uniqueness, coherent in their evolutions, calibrated for the goal to reach. They are sacred. Thus, even if they are challenging, they give us the feeling of being in the right place at the right moment. Somehow, they make sense. Krishna and Christ are two spiritual masters. It is illuminating to look at the meaning of their names, Krishna, *Kri* - action, *shna – Shuniya*, or silence. Krishna is the one who acts through and desires silence. His approach is to be neutral, in a state of non-differentiation, and to act in that awareness. Christ, *cri* – action, *ist, isht* – destiny and belonging. Christ is the one who acts considering his belonging and his destination are interchangeable. He means and wants to be what he has always been, is, and will be throughout his mission.

To be masters of ourselves, it is vital to know why, when and how, we make decisions. The first question is what we choose. In the game of life, this is free will. Throughout history, many have been resistant to discover their unknown potential. A challenge seems necessary to awaken our virtues and values. Strangely, it is this opposition that helps unravel the subconscious egoistic methods of control and sabotage. Yogis call this resistance, *karma*. A master makes *karma* the object of his experience, transforming *karma* into *Dharma* and, in so doing, respects the role *karma* plays in mastery.

BEING A MASTER

The intensity of the relationship with the encounter is proportional to the ability to endure. All the pain, vastness, ecstasy, silence, solitude, and union we experience reach the limit when we can no longer contain it. A master first expands the horizons of tolerance and then removes them. The result is that from experience, the master has tolerance and now can tolerate all other situations. This is the most genuine form of love, practical and necessary.

Being unable to love or to be loved is, in fact, a lack of tolerance. Tolerance requires a belief in one's soul, which can endure every experience. To be tolerant, we need courage. For courage, we need grit. For grit, we need knowledge. For knowledge, we need experience. And for experience, we need spirit. Thus, when we talk about love, we add the two elements of tolerance and spirit. To have mastery of the self, the soul requires a direct relationship with the experience. Involvement in the experience is necessary to feel the spirit and act from it. By allowing the experience to reach the essence of our spirit, we can reach other's psyche. By talking to the heart, we can love anybody, while talking to the mind, we can destroy them.

Those who have the mastery of the Self love, elevate, unify others. This experience with the soul elicits true knowledge, from which grit arises, followed by resolution from the decisive will. Even if coming from pain and suffering, grit gives us the capacity to overcome adversity with persistence; and thus courage becomes the base of tolerance. Courage resides in the heart; it is our soul's strength, vast, infinite, all-loving, and tolerant. The process of mastery of the Self is simple; express our true essence, which is spirit. Masters pass on this identity through their presence, by touch, gaze, or words. They give spirit to the spirit.

Another quality of mastery is honesty, approaching an experience transparently and loyally, first with ourselves and then with others. A master acts with integrity and divinity to relate through their identity. They are noble toward themselves and others; nobility is a code of conduct to act with dignity, preventing one self's corruption. Life in the mastery of the self transforms *karma* into *dharma*. In *karma* lies the call to action, and answering this call with transparency brings beauty; the beauty is in what we deliver. The four aspects of our delivery are how we appear, how we talk, how we understand, and how we deliver. These aspects are apparent in graceful behavior, manners, and relations. When we answer this call of duty to be and not having, we become experts, masters of the Self.

A master acknowledges that nothing is perfect, only the chance available and the ability to grasp it. Earlier, we used the marriage analogy to symbolize the path of *Sadhana, Aradhana,* and *Prabhupati.* The completion, therefore the perfection, is the union. Every being is complete and perfect in itself. To experience it, we need to be that unified being. The body, the mind, and the spirit are not isolated entities, and the individual neither is of the three nor is beyond them. He is the master putting them together to become one.

The basis of our teachings is that the human is a complete expression of God, a total emanation of God, being a thorough explanation of God. Those who have mastery of the Self feel this way, see this way, talk this way, taste this way, project this way. Everything is a gift of God, and they are a gift of God to others and their environment. This is what life is, and it is prosperity.

Humbleness allows true human being nature to prevail, Mother Nature and the creative nature of the universe. Thus, humans do not need to act under the pressure of time and space but in accordance with the spirit. Now we go back and see the necessity for the first step, discipline to face resistance with compassion, betrayal with kindness. Through discipline, our life becomes fulfilled and productive, and creativity flourishes. The mind, led by the consciousness, favors the spirit and the soul and reaches a vibratory frequency connecting it to the universal mind, which guides, sustains, and expands it. The result is patience and respect for ourselves, and endless endurance.

Conditions for the Mastery

A master always is clear about depth, dimension, and direction. Depth is the capacity to go within to meet the authentic Self, sense what is below the surface not only in ourselves but also in others, and perceive reality. Rooted in the core of our being, it anchors us regardless of the circumstances or challenges. It is the faculty to tap into our inner resources of spirit through self-reflection, self-assessment, and self-renewal. Dimension is the ability to locate our self, and relate to and understand our role there. It is also the sensitivity to feel our possible expansion and range of impact. Direction is the faculty to know where to direct our life to deliver our uniqueness and serve others. Once we know our direction, our doubts reduce dramatically, so that we lose less energy in thinking. Motivated by intuition, we move from intention to commit to action. Every challenge is an opportunity to grow and excel. Seeing more facets of our Self and our personality, we come closer to our true identity. Depth, dimension, and direction establish our mission, and once we embrace it, we feel ecstasy, the continuous flow of consciousness as in a constant state of love.

Masters do not use their dimension to play games. They do not seek externally because they understand the inner reality. They know the truth and add depth and direction to their dimension. Through our yogic practice, we observe that yoga affects us physically, mentally, and energetically. Yoga mainly affects the body's involuntary functions such as breathing, heart rhythm, and blood pressure. By controlling our movements in postures, kriyas, and meditations, we stimulate the involuntary nervous system, optimizing its function and giving us conscious control of these normally automatic functions. Through the triangles created in postures and mudras, specific eye focus (dhristis), and the optic and energetic focus through visualization and imagination, we stimulate the endocrine system. The depth of the experience that results from practice over time disciplines and guides our feelings, thoughts, and desires. We are able to transcend the normal involuntary processes to conscious supervision with the application of creative intelligence affecting the associative neuronal thought processes. Thus, it makes aware the involuntary physiological and mental functions. Mastery is the antithesis of unconscious action, and it transforms the human from intentional wanting to intentional action.

In *Discipline*, *Sadhana* and *Aradhana*, we saw how Kundalini Yoga's technology creates the conditions to be ourselves and express it in harmony with all of creation. Now in *Prabhupati*, we focus on decision and action. Our actions finalize the expression of Self in harmony with the creation – remembering that we are both the perfect creation and Creator of the creative process, concretely the circumstances and their source. Karmically chosen challenges provide potential to the manifestation of our being, our essence, which is the goal of mastery. This is the resurrection of the spirit.

CREATE CREATIVITY FROM THE ESSENCE OF BEING

There is no conception without perception. Then the question is, what is the source of perception. We need to understand how the Creator has created the creatures and the entire creation from himself. Before the Creator decided to create, there was nothing, an indefinite empty space, a constant and perpetual *Maha Samadhi*. If the pure creative potential is a vacuum, then there is potentially everything in a vacuum. The vacuum is both infinite non-existence and creative potential. Non-existence is the source of existence – from silence to sound, from stasis to vibratory frequency. It is in *shuniya*, with no time, no space, and no preconceptions, only with infinite compassion to relate to reality that life is born. The human goes from being a divine creation to a divine creator. Then one is complete because the Infinite being and finite expression become one. The marriage in *Aradhana* is finalized in *Prabhupati*. Kundalini Yoga science, including Humanology and the influence of Sikh tradition, are components of a non-dualistic perspective, which bases the creative human reality on the universal condition of *shuniya*, a sacred internal space from which every relation, intent, and action is possible and integrated into the cosmic design.

When we are no longer dualistic and a master of our Self, instead of trying to be liked or loved, we reflect beauty and love directly from our infinite soul's essence. If there is no duality, there is only one fact, that human beings and God are one identity. From this condition, we welcome every situation in the same way. There is no good or bad. We accept every situation neutrally to manifest our essence. In the mastery of the Self, the self's expressive power comes from the condition of non-thought, of nonbeing. When we relate to what happens from an undifferentiated state, the spirit prevails and intuitively follows the diagonal for our destiny and soul's intention. Applying intelligence to our intuition, we align our internal intention with our external projection, unblocking the subconscious conflicts and restoring the flow of *praana*, thus sustaining the neutral state and achieving the objective. As the *pranic* energy coincides with the flow of existence, our attitude and consciousness change, freeing our power to express our essence to act in integrity. When opposites integrate, their effectiveness is multiplied. For example, when *apana* and *praana* come together at the navel center, they generate *Tapa*, the psychic force of purification which, descending to the first chakra, unlocks the stored kundalini energy, so it rises in the *Sushumna*. With the necessary *praana*, one transcends limitations to discern reality from illusion. In mastery, we consciously use the facets of our personality instead of reacting from the subconscious's pressure.

Shuniya, driven by compassion rather than passion and desire, allows such mastery, the art of creating creativity from an unconditioned state, conferring originality without attachment. Without *shuniya*, instead of creative originality, we take from the past or speculate about the future, creating a false reality. The urge to create is equal in both cases, but the motivation, process, attitude, and result are diametrically opposite. The zero of *shuniya* neutralizes the polarities of existence and non-existence so that it may manifest. *Shuniya* is the gate to reality and its co-creator. In *shuniya*, the purification of love from the wedding of *Aradhana* happens, objections and opinions are lost, and the marriage of *Prabhupati* occurs. In this state of zero, we acknowledge the ego dynamics and the intellect's functioning. We conquer the mind, know our true self and express it creatively. Those who obtain this mastery, perceiving the dynamics of the universe and recognizing that they are an inseparable part of it, can guide others in the process to mastery.

The Transition

In the process of transforming from a finite human being to an infinite nature, we go through different mental and consciousness states. The soul's frequency slowly rises as the hold of the subconscious diminishes. We begin to consider new creative questions: Why have I come to this life in this environment, space, time, and circumstances? What is my uniqueness? What is my destination? There is no life without purpose.

However, we tend to try to understand through our intellect. At some point in this investigation, many look at their relationship to their family of origin, especially parents. Some people spend their entire life probing the effect of their parent's behavior, and in this search, never recover their true Self. They spend their lives either trying to be different from their parents or trying to meet their parents' expectations. Those committed to transforming stop researching the past and begin searching within to discover who they really are. The question is no longer about what their parents did in the past, but rather who they are and how to act in relation to their consciousness. They live in the present, seeing the opportunities in the challenges to their goal. Living a life in which the spirit prevails is a life of prosperity. To prosper is to overcome the adverse circumstances of time and space and bring forth an infinite abundance of possibilities. The power of transformation is to be present in the here and now of where we are, at the very moment something happens. We can learn from the past, which does not leave behind energy or reality, but rather consequences to be dealt with today. When we understand that what remains is just an impression of yesterday in the senses' memory, we can transform them today. The past is history, the present, reality, the future, imagination. In mastery, we acknowledge the past as an expression of what was done that is reflected in our reputation, the present an area in which we act, and the future as the expression of our grace.

The shift is from trying to understand to being in relation with the present environment and others – going from understanding to experimenting. Self-observation drives our transformation to become a master. Through this crystallization, the creativity of the soul becomes productive. We confront our experience from truth to unify the finite self and its instinct with the infinite Self and embrace ourselves' totality. We use our consciousness's virtues and values – patience, tolerance, and kindness to connect to the intensity of the experience. Over time, when carefully applied, the intellect and its intelligence can compute situations and find solutions to problems. Alternately, our consciousness can perceive in advance and avoid problems. Our intelligence works on behalf of our consciousness, not the other way around. Intelligence is manipulative, while consciousness never betrays us. The less conscious we are, the more we create suffering. As we transform and use more consciousness, we become intuitive. Through intuition, we perceive in a straightforward manner what it is and might be in the future or has been in the past, without intellectual, analytical, and rational thinking. Thus in the mastery of the mind, we direct our lives intuitively, consider circumstances and weigh actions with wisdom by keeping a constant relationship with our Self, others, and the environment.

Thinking takes time, and to be successful, we need to be a step ahead of time. Human actions are perfect just when they are intuitive, while continuous thinking consumes human resources, distracting us from the trinity's reality: the subject, the object, and the unknown. The unknown is everywhere at all times and is the one that really acts. We know the unknown only intuitively through silence. Through the vacuum created with silence, God's intuitive impulse dispenses impulsiveness to those who live through impulse and intuition to those who live through intuition. This is the actual activity of the master: to bring the unknown in the known. It started in *Sadhana* when the finite is acknowledged and then in *Aradhana* when the infinite, the unknown come together with the finite and known self. Now in *Prabhupati*, a gate to the unknown eases the way to mastery. A master feels and perceives reality and translates it for others. Thus, through the ages, masters have guided humanity. Through the realization of the Self, the finite human perceives the infinite pulse, inspires and attracts others to it.

THE EXPERIENCE OF LOVE

We can exist without living, make love without merging, practice yoga without ecstasy, know without knowing, and act without delivering. This existence depletes our energy; however, the inner emptiness may awaken us to our destiny. In mastery, with devotion and dedication, we embrace the duality of non-existence and bring our divinity into existence, embracing our complete and unique being while interacting with everyone and everything. With the knowledge of both our mind and the universal mind, we start living. God is pure creativity, and the power moving the creative action is love.

Love is the motivation for people to free themselves from ignorance and attain mastery of Self. Human beings, in their creative projection, created the concept of God. Love is the creative power to do the impossible. Love stops us from doing what we have always done, reacting as we have always reacted, and instead being who we truly are. The impossible becomes possible. Love allows others to express their authentic selves. Through love, we transform the limited human condition that resolves the impermanence of earthly life. By sharing this knowledge with others, we fulfill our purpose in this life. To sacrifice the unconscious, conscious and subconscious paradigms in favor of the supreme consciousness is love in action. We experience the ecstasy of the Self, existing in the beginning, now, and forever. Mastery and love have a shared purpose of absorbing and integrating the unknown's unmanifested vastness with the manifested limitation of the known. Merged in love, each action is an expression of the Self in the gentle and powerful pulse of existence, the universe's expansion and contraction.

Kriya Hypnotize Your Inner Being

September 20, 1989

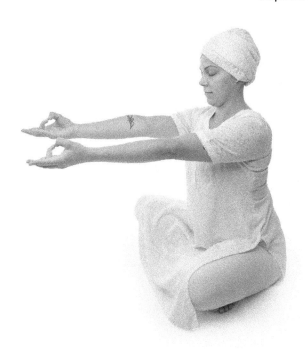

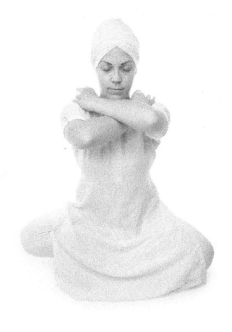

PART ONE

Time: 10 Minutes

Sit in easy pose with a straight spine, extend both arms out straight forward from the shoulders, parallel to the floor and to each other with a 90 degrees angle at the armpit, palms facing up. Place the hands in Ravi Mudra (tip of the thumbs and ring fingers touch). Gently close your eyes and concentrate at the third eye. Imagine your body as hard as steel. Let all thoughts go.

After 6 minutes start playing soft music 'I am Thine, in mine, myself …'.

PART TWO

Time: 9 Minutes

Continue listening to the music and meditating on the third eye. Slowly bend the elbows crossing the left arm over the right and bring the hands to the opposite shoulders, keep the same mudra. Raise the elbows up to point forward, upper arms are parallel to the ground.

After 3 minutes maintain the posture and come into prayer. The stress within your organs will relax, healing through your hypnotic prayer.

After additional 3 minutes Maintain the posture and change the music to *'The only education that I want, is to learn to serve you better…'* by Nirinjan Kaur.

To End. Music stops. Inhale deep and hold tight, 20 seconds. Exhale. Inhale deep, hold 20 seconds. Exhale. Inhale deep and hold it tight, 7 seconds; inhale a little more, and a little more, hold, 30 seconds. Exhale and relax.

Comments: The goal of Kundalini Yoga is to relieve the pain that comes from persistent thoughts that take us away from our true Self. It allows us to become sovereign and fulfilled, giving us the capacity to have a complete relationship with our mind and its eighty-one facets. This relationship is key to our happiness by fulfilling our destiny

Kriya Beaming and Creating the Future

June 12, 1990

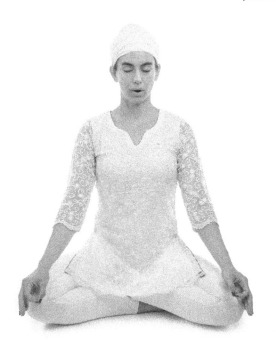

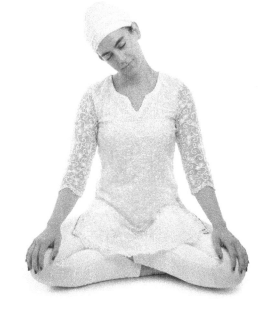

PART ONE

Time: 14 Minutes

Sit in any meditative pose with spine straight. Eyes closed. Breathe quickly through the mouth like a pipe, drinking the breath, full breath in one stroke. Exhale quickly through the nose.

End: Inhale deep, breathe normally. Immediately begin Part two.

PART TWO

Time: 24 Minutes

Eyes closed, meditate on zero, *shuniya*.

Hypnotize yourself. mentally repeat, "I am zero, my disease is zero, everything is zero". Zero applied to your thoughts and feelings of doubt and insecurity results in zero.

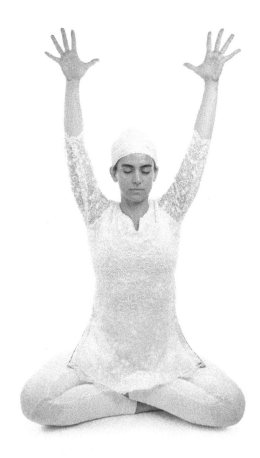

After 7 minutes, let all your negativity expand. Multiply it by zero.

After additional 4 minutes, think of what you need the most in your life. Find one word – health, work, stability, whatever it may be. Focus on it, mentally repeat it, beaming it to the universe.

End. Inhale deep, suspend, circle the head. (15s) Exhale fast. Inhale, suspend, move the neck, move the shoulders. (10s) Exhale. Inhale, suspend, keep on moving, move the entire physical spine and the body. (15s) Relax.

2 minutes, stretch arms up with fingers wide open, breathe deep and keep stretching.

End. Inhale deep, suspend (10s) inhale little more (10s), inhale little more (10s), relax.

Comments: The essence of communication is not in the words, but rather in other clues. Humans are not good listeners. We can use self-hypnosis as a tool to speak and act knowing the sequence and resultant consequences.

Meditative Kriya for Harmonious Action

February 27, 1992

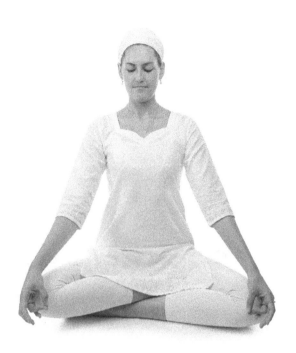

PART ONE

Time: 12 Minutes

Sit in easy pose like a yogi.

Look at the tip of the nose. Snap the fingers with thumb and Sun Finger (ring finger), arms straight. Playing 'Har Singh, Nar Singh, Neel Narayan'.

For the last 90 seconds add breath of fire.

To End: Inhale deep, relax. Immediately begin Part Two.

PART TWO

Time: 3 Minutes

Hit shoulders rhythmically with hands as hard as you can. Playing 'Wahe Guru, Sat Naam Sat Naam Ji'.

Immediately begin Part Three.

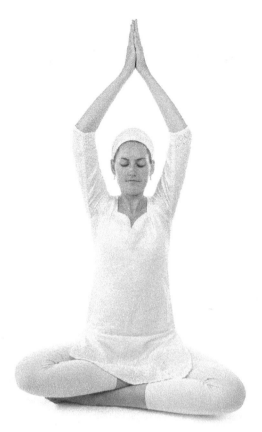
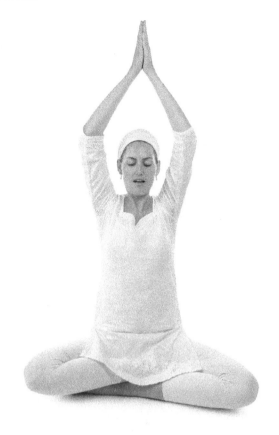

PART THREE

Time: 9.5 Minutes

Raise the arms over the head, palms together, elbows bent.

Breath deep, long and as slow as possible.

Eyes at the Tip of the Nose or closed.

For the last 2 minutes, chant 'Har, Har, Har' from the navel.

To End: Inhale deep, suspend, stretch yourself. (10s) Relax.

Comment: In the Aquarian Age, there is nothing to learn, we must have the experience. The body requires nourishment, mind requires control, soul requires strength, and they must act harmoniously. We achieve this with discipline, grace and courage.

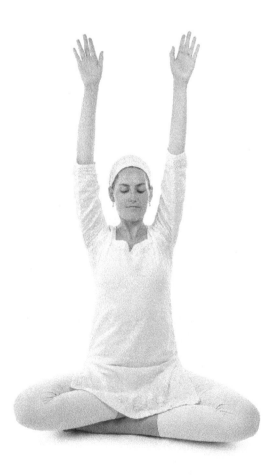

Trivani Kriya

February 29, 1992

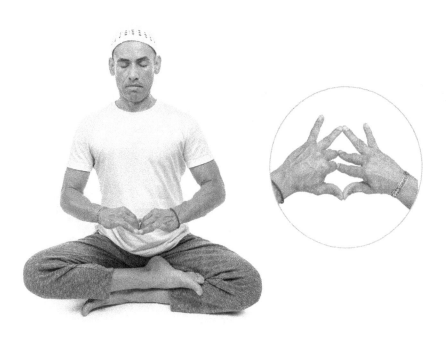

PART ONE

Time: 59 Minutes

Sit in Easy Pose with a straight spine. Bend the elbows with forearms parallel to the ground at the level of the Solar Plexus. Touch the tips of the thumbs, Jupiter Fingers (index fingers), Saturn Fingers (middle fingers) and Sun Fingers (ring fingers) together. Fingers are straight, thumbs point toward the Solar Plexus, Jupiter and Saturn fingers point down. Sun fingers, parallel to the ground, point away from the body. Mercury Fingers (pinky fingers) are free and angled higher than the Sun Fingers.

Focus the eyes at the Tip of the Nose. Breathe very slowly, longest and deepest breath, average 3 times per minute.

After 4 minutes, play "Chattr Chakkr Varti" by Kulwant Singh, just listen, let the inner hammer take care of you. Continue for 55 minutes.

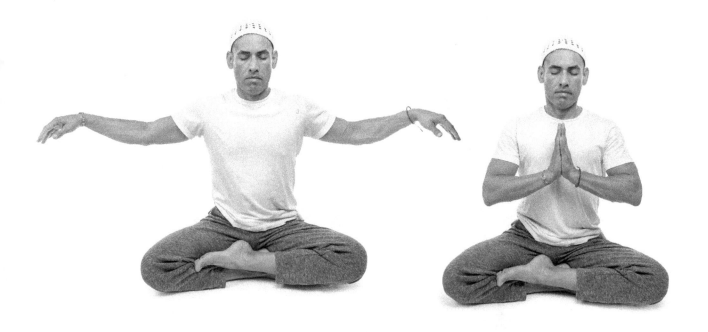

PART TWO

Time: 3 Minutes

Continue to breathe long and deep. Open the arms out to the sides, shoulder height, like wings. Slowly move the arms and hands like wings, approximately 12 inches (30 cm) up and down from the shoulder. Elbows relaxed. Create a rhythm. Move gently with the music. Continue for 3 minutes.

To End: Slowly bring the hands to Prayer Pose at the Heart Center, palm to palm, finger to finger, just touch, no force. 30 seconds. Music ends. Relax.

PART THREE

Time: 5 Minutes

Relax, take a break. Move the body a little bit. Continue for 5 minutes.

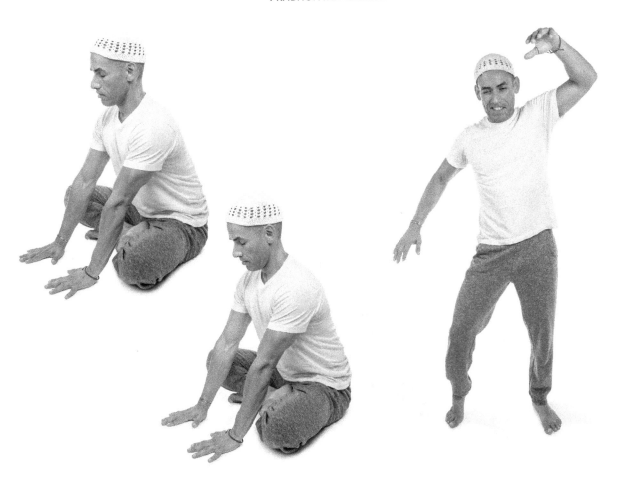

PART FOUR

Time: 5 Minutes

Sit in Easy Pose with a straight spine. Place both hands on the ground in front of the legs, bend forward slightly at the waist, elbows straight, palms flat. Put weight on the hands, chin up. Hold the posture still. Sit in a graceful, royal way. Close the eyes. Play "Har Singh, Nar Singh" by Nirinjan Kaur. Just listen, the posture will do everything. Continue for 5 minutes.

To End: Inhale deep, hold tight, put all the weight of the body on the hands as powerfully as possible. 20 seconds. Exhale. Repeat 2 more times, the last time, feel the center of the Earth in the palms of the hands.

PART FIVE

Time: 17 Minutes

Stand up. Play Punjabi Drums. Dance. Move the hands and arms, the armpits must open to regenerate the nervous system. Pick a partner, face each other and continue to dance. Continue for 17 minutes.

Comments: Dance for your health, no other reason. It needs to be a wild dance; the whole body must sweat.

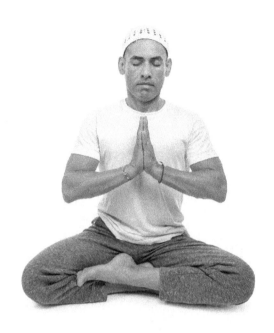

PART SIX

Time: 19 Minutes

Sit is Easy Pose with a straight spine. Place the hands in Prayer Pose at the Heart Center. Close the eyes.

Concentrate by physical force, let the breath come under control. Play "Waah Yantee, Kaar Yantee" by Nirinjan Kaur. Deeply meditate on the sound current and sing with the mantra:

WAAH YANTEE, KAAR YANTEE,

JAGADOOTPATEE, AADAK IT WHAA-HAA,

BRAHMAADAY TRAYSHAA GUROO

IT WHAA-HAY GUROO

To End: Music ends. Inhale deep, hold tight, make a prayer between you and whatever you believe in. 20 seconds. Exhale. Inhale deep, hold the breath and pray to your breath, to give you life, power, happiness, Infinity, God, whatever you want. The greatest ally of life is breath of life. 20 seconds. Exhale with a prayer. Inhale deep again, hold it and feel happy, mentally, spiritually and physically. 15 seconds. Exhale.

Comments: Your mind serves you. You must gain control of your mind. Begin now.

Meditation for the Shashra

March 4, 1992

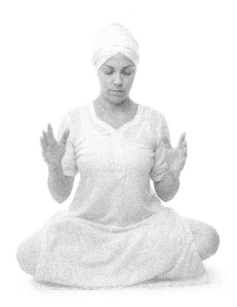
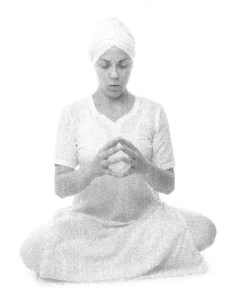

Time: 35 Minutes

Sit in easy pose with a straight spine. Focus the eyes at the tip of nose. Place the tips of the fingers together in front of the Heart Center, fingers face forward and leave space between the palms, elbows stay relaxed at the sides. Tilt the head forward with the chin toward the notch of the collarbone. Inhale deeply through the nose and move the hands apart shoulder width. Bring the fingertips back together and exhale powerfully through the mouth, blow the air through the space formed by the Jupiter Fingers (index fingers) and thumbs. Create a rhythm.

After 5 minutes, Play instrumental music softly. Indian flute and tabla music was played in class.

To End: Hold tight and raise the arms overhead, hands in Prayer Pose, lock the thumbs, elbows straight. Stretch up. 15 Seconds. Exhale. Inhale deep, stretch up, 10 seconds. Exhale. Inhale deep, hold 5 seconds. Exhale. Inhale again very deep, hold tight stretch up, 20 seconds. Cannon fire breath out, all the way out, hold the breath out, 5 seconds. Relax. Immediately eat cantaloupe to recuperate.

Comments: A basic human problem is to be concerned about the outer environments – is my job secure, do I have a nice house – and ignore caring for the self by daily nurturing and restoring the body, mind and soul. First value the gift of this life and then it will benefit those around you.

Meditation to Touch Inner Feelings

March 24, 1992

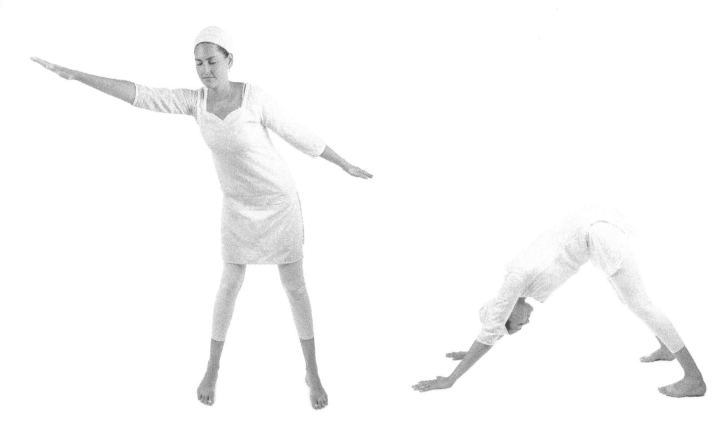

PART ONE

Time: 7 Minutes

Stand up, stretch arms diagonally 60 degrees, right in front and left behind, put the weight towards right as flying diagonally. Bend from the waist. Eyes closed. Think anything negative, wrong.

Immediately begin Part Two.

PART TWO

Time: 3 Minutes

Come into Triangle Pose, distribute weight equally on your hands and feet, relax the body.

Comments: Less weight on your hands, it is not good for your heart. If the discomfort is too much come out of the posture.

Immediately begin Part Three.

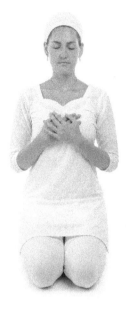
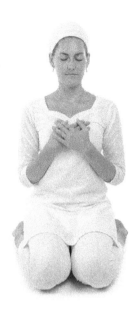
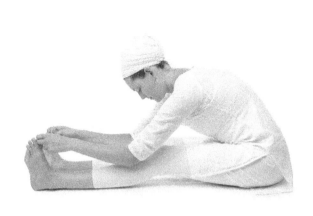

PART THREE

Time: 17 ½ Minutes

Sit in Rock Pose (if possible, sit in Celibate Pose) it will stimulate pituitary. Eyes closed, hands on the Heart Center. Sit straight, with a light Neck Lock. Feel you are in the presence of the Infinite. Be humble and divine.

After 2.5 minutes start chanting with 'Humee Hum Brahm Hum' (Nirinjin Kaur) playing.

Immediately begin Part Four.

PART FOUR

Time: 5 Minutes

Stretch legs forward, bend forward and hold your big toes. Close your eyes and meditate, let yourself go, take a nap. Music continues.

After 3 minutes change music start playing 'Happiness, happiness, Nobility, Infinity'

End. Inhale, suspend the breath, squeeze yourself tight as steel. (20s) Cannon fire exhale. Repeat two more times. Relax.

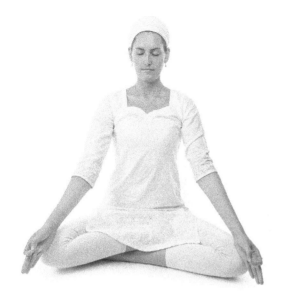

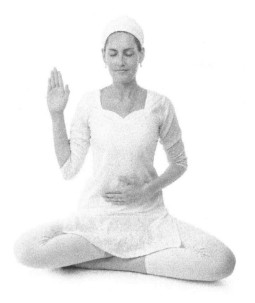

PART FIVE

Time: 9 Minutes

Come into Easy Pose, eyes closed, meditate.

Continue to imagine that you face to face with God. You are not inferior; the Infinite is within you; talk with each other.

After 3 minutes start playing 'Meditation whole creation...' by Wahe Guru Kaur. Immediately begin Part Six.

PART SIX

Time: 8.5 Minutes

Continue playing the music. Place the left hand on the navel, fingers point to the right, right hand held as if taking an oath, fingers together. Meditate.

For the last 1.5 minutes, hypnotize yourself and imagine your spine as a tube of light. As you receive praana, the life force, your spine becomes brighter and you become brighter, more youthful and beautiful.

End. Inhale deep, exhale.

Comments: The change from the Piscean to the Aquarian Age signifies a change in the earth's electromagnetic field. If we are not able to change our frequency, we may survive, but physically and mentally we may be lost. We must generate inner vitality, so that our brain can process this change. Otherwise, you become sad about the past and afraid of the future. We have the capacity to stop, to pause in stillness. In *shuniya*, we surrender as at an altar. In the zero, in that emptiness, everything effortlessly comes to you.

Kriya to Cross the Electromagnetic Field

March 25, 1992

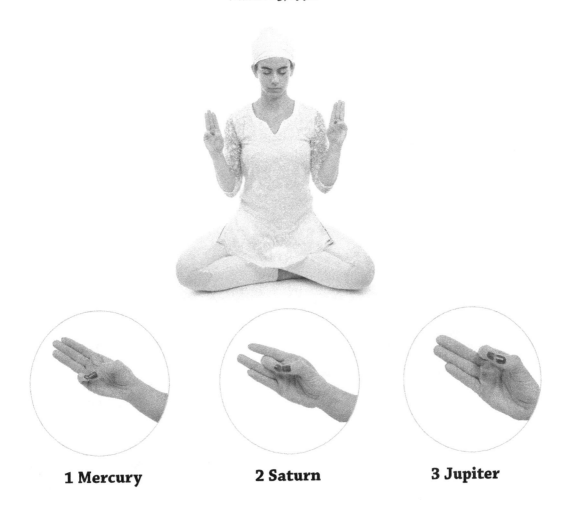

1 Mercury   **2 Saturn**   **3 Jupiter**

Time: 5+14 Minutes

PART ONE

Time: 5 Minutes

Sit in Easy Pose with a straight spine. Bend the elbows, hands are near the shoulders, palms face forward. Upper arms are relaxed near the body. Create a sequence; touch the tips of the Mercury Fingers (pinky fingers) and the thumb tips together; touch the tips of the Saturn Fingers (middle fingers) and thumb tips together; touch the tips of the Jupiter Fingers (index fingers) and

thumb tips together. Continue this sequence at your own rate, beginning with Buddhi Mudra (Mercury finger and thumb tips) with each cycle. Look at the Tip of the Nose.

After 2 minutes, Raise the knees each time the finger tips touch, lower them as the mudra changes. Keep the same rhythm. Continue for 3 more minutes.

Comments: Remember the thumb touches every finger, except the Ring Finger. For the best results move quickly

281

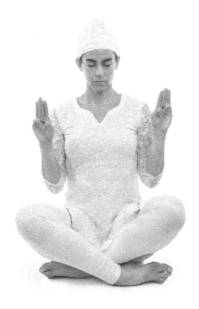
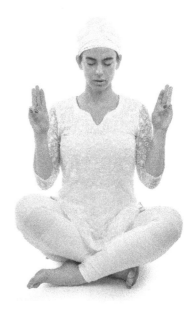

PART TWO

Time: 14 Minutes

Continue the mudra and knee movement. Chant HUMEE HUM BRAHM HUM in monotone with the tip of the tongue on the middle of the upper palate to experience the sound differently. Play the mantra music by Nirinjan Kaur. Coordinate the movement of the fingers and the knees with the sound current. Continue for 14 minutes.

To End: Inhale deep, hold the breath. Synchronize the body, including the inside of the skull, tighten it. 25 seconds. Exhale. Inhale deep, hold that posture very nicely and tighten it. From the top to the bottom go slowly down the body, bring everything to *shuniya*, zero until you feel it in your toes. 25 seconds. Exhale. Inhale deep, hold your breath and bring the body to *shuniya* from top to bottom. It's a very good adjustment, go down all the way till you reach your toes. 30 seconds. Exhale, relax. Talk to each other for 1 minute to become human again.

Comments: When we are in self-denial, we attack others. We are not happy and have no gratitude. To be grateful, we need first to feel that we are great and remember that we are made in the likeness of God. Then we feel full, whole. When we deny our greatness, we search outside to fill our perceived lack, we seek comfort from things and from people. We become insensitive to ourselves and others. Happiness comes in knowing ourselves, and not denying the Self.

Meditation for Communication

March 28, 1992

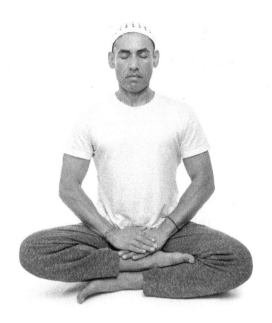

PART ONE

Time: 1 Minute

Sit in Easy Pose with a straight spine. Place the left hand in the lap with the right hand on top, both palms face down. Press down on the hands like a weight from the elbows and shoulders, keep the chest lifted. Close the eyes.

Speak these three words: RATI, ROTI, RETI. Say RATI and imagine that you are imperial, like a king or queen. Say ROTI and imagine a huge table of 36 edibles and the satisfaction of its beauty. Say RETI and imagine the action of cutting or filing something smooth. One cycle takes 5 seconds.

Comment: This is a practice working with the *naad*, the science of sound. Repetition of each sound with an image creates a personal experience. Each person has an individual experience, different from each other. Thus, in conversation, speak so that the other person understands you, not for your own satisfaction. Listen deeply and then you speak with universal wisdom. This is the meaning of the line from Japji: *Suniai sidh peer sur nath*.

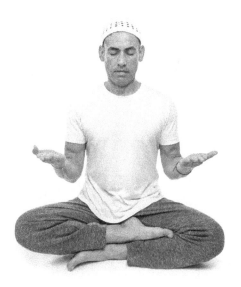
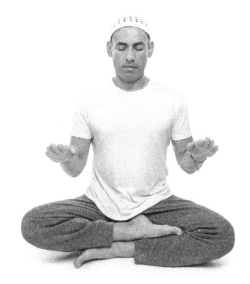
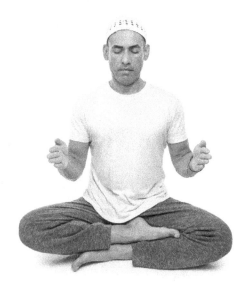
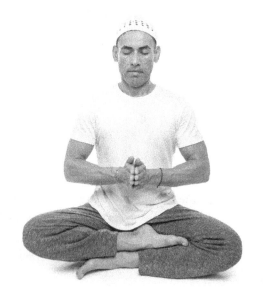

PART TWO

Time: 14 Minutes

Remain in Easy Pose with a straight spine.
Bend the elbows, keep them relaxed by the body,
forearms forward, palms face up, fingers together,
thumbs relaxed. Move the hands in the following
sequence, move from the wrist with precision:

1- palms face up.

2- palms face down.

3- palms apart facing each other.

4- palms meet in the center.

5- palms apart facing each other.

6- palms face down.

7- palms face up to begin again.

Count out loud in sequence. After 3 minutes,
randomly change the sequence.

Comments: This is best practiced in the classroom
with a teacher to guide the sequencing. When you
do this exercise at home mentally speak your own
numbers and listen and correct yourself on it.

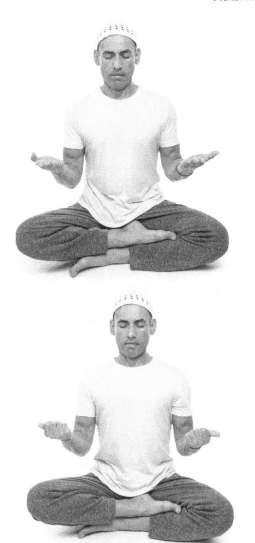

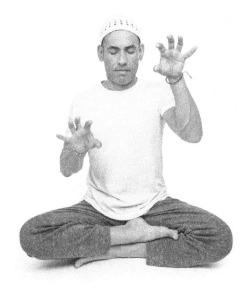

PART THREE

Time: 6 Minutes

Remain in Easy Pose with the forearms forward, elbows relaxed, palms face up. Open and close the fingers into the palms as fast as possible. Thumbs are relaxed.

Look at the Tip of the Nose.

To End: Inhale deep. Immediately begin Part Four.

Comments: caution, in this *tattva* stimulating exercise, if there is any head discomfort, stop the posture.

PART FOUR

Time: 5 Minutes

Remain in Easy Pose. Bend the fingers like claws, move the hands in a small circular motion in front of the body as if scratching at something. Move very fast.

Hold the front teeth together.

To End: Inhale, immediately begin Part Five.

Comments: Don't be gentle. The faster the motion, the better the result.

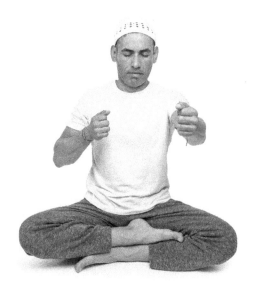

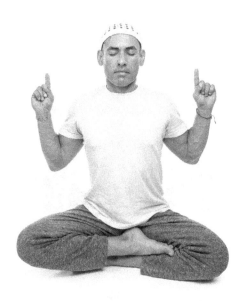

PART FIVE

Time: 8 Minutes

Remain in Easy Pose. Lock the back molars, keep them tight together. Make fists with both hands and alternately punch straight forward from the shoulders. Move quickly and powerfully.

To End: Inhale, immediately begin Part Six.

Comments: Tremendous pressure on the elbows will take care of the digestive system. Hit hard with a sense of victory.

PART SIX

Time: 24 Minutes

Remain in Easy Pose. Extend the Jupiter Fingers (index fingers) straight, hold the rest of the fingers down with the thumbs. Palms face forward. Bend the elbows, forearms perpendicular to the ground, parallel to each other. Shoulders back, chest out. Do not let the hands fall forward. Look at the Tip of the Nose.

Breathe slowly, 4 breaths a minute. 5 seconds to breathe in, 5 seconds to hold, 5 seconds to breathe out.

After 3 minutes, play 'Heal my world'.

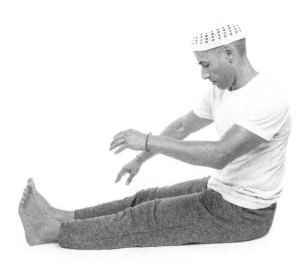

To End: Inhale deep, music stops, hold the breath. 10 seconds. Exhale. Inhale, hold 5 seconds. Exhale. Inhale, hold tight, synchronize the body, 10 seconds. Exhale, relax. Move the shoulders and body, stretch out, play "Bountiful, Beautiful", loudly. **2-10 minutes**.

Comments: When we gradually change our inner then the outer will also change. This is the inverse of what we tend to believe. If God is everywhere, God is within us. When we acknowledge that God is within us, we no longer are alone. Listening to God within, to God that is everywhere, we can move through life without drama.

To be happy in this play of life, we experience life beyond duality and polarities. When we know ourselves and our infinity, we act from that vastness. We are no longer the doer, but the witness, the being. Communication from this space of self-acceptance brings the wisdom of the universe.

Meditation for Vitality

September 4, 1991

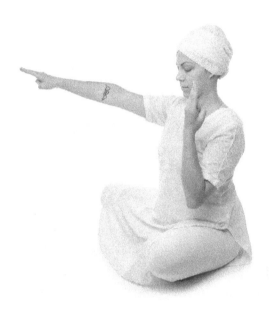

PART ONE

Time: 10 Minutes

Sit in Easy Pose with a straight spine. Lock the Sun Fingers (ring fingers) and Mercury Fingers (pinky fingers) down with the thumbs. Extend the Jupiter Fingers (index fingers) and Saturn Fingers (middle fingers) straight and together on both hands.

Raise the right arm just above shoulder height to keep the armpit open, bring it out 60 degrees from the center of the body. Keep the elbow straight, bend the wrist with the palm facing forward.

Bend the left arm keeping the elbow against the rib cage and bring the hand to shoulder height,

palm facing the body, forearm perpendicular to the ground. Balance the arms. Focus the eyes on the Tip of the Nose. Hypnotize yourself... Eliminate your physical body and turn yourself into thirty trillion white light, dancing cells. Breathe very, very long and slowly.

To End: Inhale deep, hold tight, bring both hands on your chest. Exhale. Immediately begin Part Two.

Comments: Keep the elbow straight to support the circulatory system. Holding the arm at sixty degree, supports the parasympathetic nervous system.

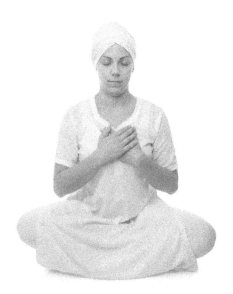

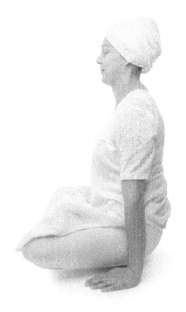

PART TWO

Time: 11 Minutes

Remain in Easy Pose. Keep both hands on the Heart Center. Press the Heart Center hard on the inhale, release the pressure on the exhale. Breathe very deep, slowly and calmly.

After 1 minute, Continue the posture. Play 'Ang Sang Wahe Guru' by Nirinjin Kaur softly. Continue for 9 minutes.

To End: Inhale deep hold for 20 seconds. Make your entire body like steel, synchronize, Pratyahara. Exhale. Repeat 2 more times. Then relax and immediately talk to another person for 1 minute.

Comments: This exercise clears your subconscious and its hidden agendas. It will increase your vitality.

PART THREE

Time: 5 minutes

Remain in Easy Pose with a straight spine. Put the hands on the floor next to the hips. Lift and drop the body very fast.

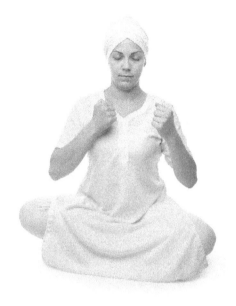

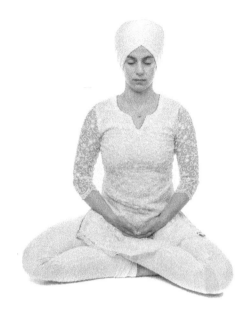

PART FOUR

Time: 5 minutes

Make fists with both hands. Alternately beat the chest with the fists. Hit fast and hard.

After 3 minutes, begin Breath of Fire. Continue for 2.5 minutes.

To End: Inhale, hold the breath, continue to beat the chest; 10 seconds, inhale more, hold tight and continue to beat the chest; 10 seconds. Relax.

Comments: This posture will stimulate the metabolism. It is a good daily practice for the glandular system to support our health

PART FIVE

Time: 2 minutes

In Easy Pose, relax the hands in the lap and interlace the fingers with the thumbs touching. Eyes focus on the tip of the nose. Meditate and Chant: HUMEE HUM BRAAHM HUM

Comments: Human life has a light, a radiance. We are bright when we have vitality. We choose to live a simple life - healthy, happy and holy. We consciously choose how we live; we choose what we take in and what we release; we choose what we see, hear, eat and drink, what we receive intuitively and what we say and project. Our light can take away our inner darkness and that of others.

GLOSSARY

Aad: the primary creativity. The original Being.

Abhyasa: Sanskrit word meaning "practice" towards a peaceful mind.

Adi Mantra: "Ong Namo Guroo Dev Namo", the mantra repeated at least times before every class or practice of Kundalini Yoga.

Ahangkar: One of the Impersonal Minds. He transcendental ego, the fundamental principle active in nature and mind that creates boundaries, identity, and attachment to things. It creates the sense of "me and mine" which is considered a fundamental tendency in the evolution of complexity and differentiation of objects and thoughts in the universe.

Ajapa Japa: The effortless repetition of a mantra, so that the words become deeply realized.

Akashic Record: The memory of the entire existence of the universe, every thought, word and action, all information and knowledge from the beginning of time and forever.

Amrit Vela: Literally, the ambrosial hours. The first hours of the morning, about two and a half hours before sunrise. A special time when you are most receptive to the soul and can clear the subconscious of wrong habits. It is considered the optimum time to practice a *Sadhana*.

Ang Sang Wahe Guru: The realization that no part of us, no action taken, nothing in life is not a part of the Infinite vibration. We are one.

Apana: One of the five vayus in the body, abiding below the navel with a downward movement and governing the functions of elimination.

Applied Intelligence or Applied Mind: Simply wisdom. When the 3 functional minds – negative, positive and neutral are under your psyche which allows you to focus and respond automatically and effectively with intuition, intelligence and comprehensive comparative

Aquarian Age: The current astrological age, starting in 2012. This age will witness a radical change in consciousness, human sensitivity and technology, requiring a new relationship to the mind.

Arc line: In yogic anatomy, one of the ten bodies. The arc of light, halo, that goes from one ear to the other. It reflects the interaction of the soul of the person with its vital energy resources and reflects the potential, destiny and health of the person. The female body has a second arc line, going from a nipple to nipple.

Asana: Literally position or seat; a yogic posture. One of patanjali's Eight Limbs of Yoga.

Ashram: A learning center for spiritual growth, in which people live together in community. In ancient Indian texts, one of four age-based life stages to happiness and liberation.

Ashtang: Literally means eight limbed. Used for mantras with eight beats.

Baisakhi or Vaisakhi: A historical and religious festival. Culturally it celebrates the start of the month of Vaisakha and the spring harvest festival. For Sikhs, it commemorates the day when Guru Gobind Singh, the tenth Sikh Guru, founded the Khalsa order, the "Pure ones", in 1699.

Bana: The form, the way a Khalsa dresses, as indicated by Guru Gobind Singh, to project the highest consciousness.

Bani: The word of God included in the Holy Sikh scriptures. The sound wave keeping the mind focused on God.

Bhagavad Gita: Literally "The song of the blessed". It's a piece of high spiritual value included in the epic poem Mahabharata (chapters 25-42 of the VI book). It's considered a fundamental text of the Hindu philosophy including the concept of the Karma Yoga, the yoga of action.

Bhakta: Devotee, those who practice the Bhakti.

Bhakti: Total devotion and love to God. Devotional aspect of the yoga.

Brahman: The cosmic unity from which the creation originated.

Buddhi: One of the three Impersonal Minds. The first most etheric manifestation of the Universal Mind from which all other areas of the mind are derived. The quality or function to recognize with clarity, discernment and wisdom the real from the imaginary in the impressions which are received.

Chardi Kala: State of consciousness in which the spirit is always elevated, and the mind is focused and stable despite life's situations. A basic concept in Sikhism

Chitta: The Universal Mind, the mind that permeates all that exists in nature.It is a part of Prakriti

Chuni or Chunni: Long scarf used by Indian women to cover their head. A symbol of grace, modesty and respect.

Cycles of Life: Cycles of development, consisting of 18 year cycle of life energy, 11 year cycle of intelligence and 7 year cycle of consciousness. These cycles Like tides, these cycles pace the development of awareness, applied intelligence and our physical being. Awareness of these cycles and their balance helps us to find fulfillment.

Darshan: From the Sanskrit root "drsh", to see. Indicates the vision or contact with a Saint or the divinity.

Dharana: Focus. To focus and channel one's attention on a single object.

Dharma: A path of righteous living, both an ideal of virtue and a path of action infused with clear awareness that bring the soul in synchronicity with the universe. Action without reaction.

Dhyana: Meditation. The uninterrupted union between the mind with the object of the meditation.

Divali or Diwali: The festival of lights, one of the most important festivals in the Hindu tradition. It's celebrated during fall and symbolizes victory over the darkness, the good over the evil.

Functional Minds: The three aspects to the mind (Negative/Protective, Positive/Expansive and Neutral/Meditative) that act as guides for the personal sense of self. When all three are balanced, the mind is enlightened and able to reflect the uniqueness of the soul.

Golden Chain: Historically, the line of spiritual masters who have preceded us - the Kundalini Yoga teachers throughout the ages. Practically it is the subtle link between the consciousness of a student and the master and the teachings. This link requires the student to put aside the ego and its limitations and act in synchrony and devotion to the highest consciousness of the master and the teachings.

Gunas: The three qualities that make up the fundamental forces in nature and the mind. Their interaction give motion to the world and make up the realm of our experience. They are Sattva, Rajas and Tamas, inseparable and occurring in infinite combinations.

Guru: That which leads one from the darkness of ignorance (gu) to the light (ru). It can be a person, a teaching or in its most subtle form – the Word. Spiritual guide.

Hukam: Literally command or order. In Sikhism, Hukam represents the goal of becoming in harmony with the will of God and thus attaining inner peace. It also designates the practice of opening up at random to a page in the Sikh scripture (Siri Guru Granth Sahib) to receive God's guidance for the day or for a particular question.

Humanology: The applied science and psychology of the human psyche for the fulfillment of human potential in body, mind and spirit including practical life style guidelines, Kundalini Yoga and meditation with Shabd Guru.

Ida: One of the three main nadis in the body through which subtle energy flows, linked to the flow of praana through the left nostril and relating to lunar energy.

Impersonal Minds: The three major functions of the Universal Mind that create qualities of experience, cognition and judgment. They are Ahangkar, Buddhi and Manas. They are impersonal, since they exist independent of or before the individual sense of self.

Ishnaan (Hydrotherapy): Water-therapy, involving bathing in cold water to open and flush the capillaries, thus increasing circulation and improving the glandular system and general health of the body.

Japa: Literally to repeat. Alert, continuous and conscious repetition of a mantra.

Jaapji Sahib: An inspired poem composed by Guru Nanak that gives a view of the cosmos, the soul, the mind, the challenge in life and the impact of our actions.

Jiwan Mukta: Comes from the Sanskrit jiwan - life - and mukti - liberation. It means freed in life, the one who reaches the non attachment to Maya during his existence, as well as the highest spiritual state of union with the One.

Karma: The cosmic law of cause and effect, action and reaction.

Khalsa: Order founded by the tenth Guru, Gobind Singh. Khalsa means "the pure ones".

Krishna: Hindu deity. The eighth descent of Vishnu which marks the end of the Dvpara Yuga (the bronze age, third Hindu cosmological era). In some traditions it is considered the total incarnation of the divine.

Kriya: Literally means completed action. In the Kundalini Yoga, it relates to a sequence of postures and yogic techniques used to determine a specific impact on the psyche, body or self. These effects have been codified and elaborated by Yogi Bhajan.

Langar: One of the essential and unique aspects of Sikh tradition, a free meal for everyone, and represents Sikh values of equality and sharing.

Laya Yoga: The use of sound and mantra with rhythm and a sensitivity to its subtle structure merging the finite with the Infinite.

Lingam: Phallic symbol, revered in Shiva temples as an emblem of Shiva. Representation of the male creative energy.

Maharabharata: One of the two major Sanskrit epics of ancient India, the other being the Rāmāyana.

Manas: One of the three Impersonal functions of the Universal Mind, the sensory mind that deals with sensory impressions, sequences and desires and impulses generated from their combinations. It is the closest to what traditional western psychology relates to as the mind.

Mantra: Words and sounds that tune or control the mind. Man means mind and tra-ang is the wave or movement of the mind. The impact from the repetition of a mantra is through the movement of the tongue on the meridian points in the mouth, through the meaning of the words, through the pattern of energy and rhythm (the vibratory wave). This directly affects the chemistry of the brain and the nervous system.

Maya: The illusion of reality. The sensory experience of ourselves and the world surrounding us making us identify with the ego creating a sense of limitation and separation.

Naad: The inner sound that is subtle and all-present; the direct expression of the Infinite. The essence of all sound.

Naadi: The channels of subtle energy within the body, where the praana flows. There are said to be 72,000 with 3 major ones.

Naam: Name. It is referred to as the Word. It gives identity, form and expression to that which was subtle, the manifestation of God.

Naam Japa: Repetition of the divine Name.

Nada Brahman: transcendental sound; traditionally from the Vedic scriptures.

Patanjali: The compiler of the Yoga Sūtras or Yoga Aphorisms, a text on Yoga theory and practice, considered the foundation of classical Yoga. We know little about the actual person, he is believed to have lived between 2nd and 4th century CE.

Pauree: Literally step. A section of verse in the Sri Guru Granth Sahib, the Sikh holy scripture.

Pingala: One of the three main nadis in the body through which subtle energy flows, linked to the flow of the praana through the right nostril and related to solar energy.

Praana: The universal life force that gives motion. It regulates the modes and moods of the mind.

Pratyahara: One of the eight limbs of yoga, it is the reabsorption of the senses to synchronize the attention on a unique object. It is said that in Pratyaharaa we bring everything to zero, shuniya.

Raga: In classic Indian music, musical structures, following very specific execution rules, based on musical basic scales. Each raga has a symbolic value and it is associated with different emotions, seasons and the hours of the day.

Raja Yoga: The royal or highest path of the yoga, which leads to the spiritual realization through the mastery of every internal and external manifestation of the Self.

Rehit Maryada: Code of Conduct, guidelines about the social and religious life of a Sikh.

Rishi: A wise sage, seer, to whom after deep meditation attained spiritual knowledge.

Sadhak or Sadaka: One who practices *Sadhana*. Spiritual practitioner.

Sadhana: A spiritual discipline.

Samadhi: Complete realization. Union of the one who meditates with the object of the meditation, of the individual Self with the supreme Self.

Samskara: Subtle impressions, traces of memory, patterns of behavior brought from past lives.

Seva: Selfless service, a key principal in Sikhism.

Shabd: Sound wave, especially subtle sound imbued with consciousness. Divine word. In Sikhism a devotional hymn from the Siri Guru Granth Sahib.

Shabd Guru: The word pronounced by the Guru. The sound and words gathered in the Sikh scripture, the Siri Guru Granth Sahib.

Shakti: The creative power and energy of the universe, without it nothing can manifest. It is the feminine principle, also known as Prakriti.

Shiva: Consciousness, the masculine principle. Also known as Purusha. In the Hindu trinity including Brahma and Vishnu, Shiva is known as "The Destroyer". Revered as Yogisvara, the Lord of Yoga.

Shuniya: "Science of zero". The state of consciousness in which the constant action of thought is inhibited, the ego is reduced to zero. You do not grasp or act, Nature acts for you.

Sushumna: One of the three main nadis in the body through which subtle energy flows. It is associated to the central channel of the spine and is associated with neutrality. The path through which the kundalini energy ascends when it is awakened. Sikh: It literally means disciple or student. Those who follow the teachings of the Siri Guru Granth Sahib.

Simran: Deep meditative process in which the constant memory of the divine name is remembered without any conscious effort.

Siri Guru Granth Sahib: Holy compilation of the words of the Sikh Gurus, as well as Hindu, Muslim, Sufi and other saints. It's the expression of consciousness derived from a state of mystic union with God. It is considered the eleventh and living Guru of the Sikhs.

Vaisakhi: See Baisakhi.

Vac Siddhi: The two terms come from Sanskrit. Var means word or voice. Siddhi means power, perfection. Vac Siddhi is the power of the word, so that the word is manifested.

Veda: Sanskrit word means to know or knowledge. The ancient Hindu scriptures, said to be divine revelation.

Yoni: Sanskrit word meaning origin or source that has come to mean the female sexual organs.

About the Author

Sadhana Singh is a Kundalini Yoga Lead Trainer committed to teach and empower new teachers and future trainers in Level 1, 2, and 3 courses internationally. An inspired author, he wrote 15 books in the past three decades about the practice, discipline, and philosophy of Kundalini Yoga and its different applications in the many fields of human life.

Sadhana Singh also acts as a dedicated counselor for individuals and companies, addressing the Science of Mind and the Humanology for creativity, excellence, leadership, and success. His experience led him to develop a series of KRI Specialty Courses: "The Science of Mind and Humanology for Leadership and Success", "Guru Leadership" and "Kundalini Yoga Counseling".

From this background, he created Aequanime, a project that holds the mission to spread the yogic lifestyle, nutrition, and techniques to help people manifest their potential. All these activities are run by Anter Vidya, an institution founded by Sadhana Singh that promotes the science of essence to facilitate human expression in every facet of life.

He is also the author of *Everyday Excellence: The Art of Success*, published by Kundalini Research Institute, in 2010.

CPSIA information can be obtained
at www.ICGtesting.com
Printed in the USA
FSHW021157170521